DONALD E. NEWELL, M.D
4UU-C S.E. 131st AVE.
SUITE #306
VANCOUVER, WA 98684
(206) 256-4425

W9-DBN-517

AMERICAN ACADEMY OF OTOLARYNGIC ALLERGY

Series Editor
Jacquelynne P. Corey, M.D., F.A.C.S., F.A.A.O.A.

In Vitro Testing

Ivor A. Emanuel, M.D., F.A.A.O./HNS, F.A.A.O.A.

Private Practice
Ear, Nose, and Throat/Allergy
San Francisco, California
Clinical Assistant Professor
Department of Otolaryngology
University of California
San Francisco, California

1994

Thieme Medical Publishers, Inc. New York
Georg Thieme Verlag Stuttgart · New York

Thieme Medical Publishers, Inc.
381 Park Avenue South
New York, New York 10016

IN VITRO TESTING
Ivor A. Emanuel

Library of Congress Cataloging-in-Publication Data

In vitro testing / [edited by] Ivor A. Emanuel.
 p. cm.—(AAOA monograph series)
 Includes bibliographical references and index.
 ISBN 0-86577-521-4 (Thieme Medical).—ISBN 3-13-100221-2 (G.
Thieme Verlag)
 1. Allergy—Diagnosis. 2. Diagnosis, Laboratory.
3. Radioallergosorbent test. I. Emanuel, Ivor A. II. Series.
 [DNLM: 1. Hypersensitivity—immunology. 2. Hypersensitivity-
-diagnosis. 3. Immunoassay—methods. QW 900 I35 1994]
RC586.I53 1994
616.97'075—dc20
DNLM/DLC
for Library of Congress   94-36576
                                                                CIP

Copyright © 1994 by Thieme Medical Publishers, Inc. This book, including all parts thereof, is legally protected by copyright. Any use, exploitation or commercialization outside the narrow limits set by copyright legislation, without the publisher's consent, is illegal and liable to prosecution. This applies in particular to photostat reproduction, copying, mimeographing or duplication of any kind, translating, preparation of microfilms, and electronic data processing and storage.

Important note: Medicine is an ever-changing science. Research and clinical experience are continually broadening our knowledge, in particular our knowledge of proper treatment and drug therapy. Insofar as this book mentions any dosage or applications, readers may rest assured that the authors, editors, and publishers have made every effort to ensure that such references are strictly in accordance with the state of knowledge at the time of production of the book. Nevertheless, every user is requested to carefully examine the manufacturers' leaflets accompanying each drug to check on his own responsibility whether the dosage schedules recommended therein or the contraindications stated by the manufacturers differ from the statements made in the present book. Such examination is particularly important with drugs that are either rarely used or have been newly released on the market.

Some of the product names, patents, and registered designs referred to in this book are in fact registered trademarks or proprietary names even though specific reference to this fact is not always made in the text. Therefore, the appearance of a name without designation as proprietary is not to be construed as a representation by the publisher that it is in the public domain.

Printed in the United States of America.

5 4 3 2 1

TMP ISBN 0-86577-521-4
GTV ISBN 3-13-100221-2

· *Contents* ·

· *Contributors* ·

**Rosemary Alden, R.N., M.S.,
A.S.O.A.T.**
Director of Technical Support
Kabi Pharmacia Diagnostics
Piscataway, New Jersey

**Jack B. Anon, M.D., F.A.C.S.,
F.A.A.O.A.**
Clinical Assistant Professor
Department of Otolaryngology
University of Pittsburgh
    College of Medicine
Pittsburgh, Pennsylvania

Private Practice
Erie, Pennsylvania

Barbara Cordes, R.N.
Nurse Consultant
MRT Laboratories
Hackensack, New Jersey

Affiliate, American College
    of Allergy and Immunology

Member, American In Vitro
    Allergy and Immunology Society

**Jacquelynne P. Corey, M.D., F.A.C.S.,
F.A.A.O.A.**
Assistant Professor of Otolaryngology
University of Chicago
Pritzker School of Medicine
Chicago, Illinois

Treasurer
American Academy of Otolaryngic
    Allergy
Chicago, Illinois

Vice President, American In Vitro
    Allergy
    and Immunology Society
Chicago, Illinois

**Ivor A. Emanuel, M.D., F.A.A.O./
HNS, F.A.A.O.A.**
Clinical Assistant Professor
    Department of Otolaryngology
University of California
San Francisco, California

Fellow, American Academy of
    Otolaryngology/Head and
    Neck Surgery

Fellow,
American Academy of
    Otolaryngic Allergy

Fellow, American In Vitro
    Allergy and Immunology Society

Member, American College
    of Allergy and Immunology

AAOA Council Member
    Director of Scientific Programs

Founding Member, Secretary,
    and Board of Directors, American
    In Vitro Allergy and
    Immunology Society

Member of Editorial Board,
    International Allergy Digest
    and New Horizons in
    Otolaryngic Allergy

Private Practice
San Francisco, California

Richard Fadal, M.D.
Clinical Assistant Professor
Family Practice and Community
Medicine
The University of Texas
Southwestern Medical Center
Dallas, Texas

Matt Haus, M.D.
Honorable Secretary
Allergy Society of South Africa

Council Member
College of Medicine of South Africa
South Africa

**Hueston King, M.D., F.A.C.S.,
F.A.C.A.**
Clinical Associate Professor
Department of Otolaryngology
University of Texas
Southwestern Medical Center
Dallas, Texas

Private Practice
Venice, Florida

**William P. King, M.D., F.A.C.S.,
F.A.A.O.A.**
Clinical Assistant Professor
Department of Otorhinolaryngology
Baylor College of Medicine
Houston, TX

Private Practice
Corpus Christi, Texas

**Richard L. Mabry, M.D., F.A.C.S.,
F.A.A.O.A.**
Professor
Department of Otorhinolaryngology
University of Texas
Southwestern Medical Center
Dallas, Texas

Donald J. Nalebuff, M.D.
Associate Professor
Department of Otolaryngology
New Jersey College of
Medicine and Dentistry
Newark, NJ

Attending Physician
Holy Name Hospital
Teaneck, New Jersey

Lewis L. Perelmutter, Ph.D.
Professor
Department of Pediatrics
Thomas Jefferson University
Philadelphia, Pennsylvania

Vice President, Director of Research
Immuno Response Technology, Inc.
Berlin, New Jersey

**Maurice L. Perou, M.D., F.C.A.P.,
F.A.S.C.P.**
Pathologist and
Director of Laboratories (retired)
Community General Hospital
Sterling, Illinois

Morrison Community Hospital
Morrison, Illinois

Dixon State Hospital
Dixon, Illinois

Pathologist
Katherine Shaw Bethea Hospital
Dixon, Illinois

Consulting Pathologist
Illinois State Psychiatric Institute
Chicago, Illinois

Richard J. Trevino, M.D.
Clinical Associate Professor
Department of Otolaryngology
Louisiana State University
Shreveport, Louisiana

· *Foreword* ·

It is my pleasure to introduce the second volume of the American Academy of Otolaryngic Allergy monograph series on diagnostic *in vitro* testing. This is the first clinical textbook for physicians on the use of *in vitro* methodologies for allergy testing. This series was designed to provide reference texts for our members in all areas of otolaryngic allergy practice. As such, this volume should be immediately welcomed in our libraries, and should also prove an invaluable reference for other allergists, family practitioners, internists, and pediatricians interested in learning about the topic. It should be a "must" for the reference library of all clinical pathologists, laboratory directors, Ph.D.s, clinical consultants, technical and general laboratory supervisors, and medical technologists/technicians concerned with operating a diagnostic *in vitro* laboratory.

Jacquelynne P. Corey, M.D.

· *Introduction* ·

It is timely that the publication of this manual on *in vitro* allergy testing occurs exactly 100 years after the introduction of the first human inoculation of diphtheria antitoxin, in 1894. This event marked the beginning of a period of intense investigation into the immune system, especially in the areas of hyperimmune states and allergy, only to be rivaled by the discovery of the immunoglobulins many years later.

Shortly after the first injection of the antitoxin horse serum, it was noted that violent reactions and sudden death could follow. At that time, the exact nature of the reaction was not understood other than that the deaths always occurred following the primary injection.

In 1916, Robert Cooke, writing in the *Journal of Immunology*, noted the similarity between peculiar drug reactions and other reactions from foreign proteins in specifically hypersensitive persons, and realized that they were "allergic reactions." It was in this paper that reference was first made to the fact that these reactions could take place when an allergen was introduced into an individual by a diagnostic skin test (mostly intradermal), and subcutaneous or intravenous injections. Cooke also called attention to the danger of constitutional reactions from therapeutic injections, especially pollen extracts.

Until this article, no one had seriously considered the important relationship of constitutional reactions to, and as a consequence of, diagnostic skin testing and the therapeutic injections for hypersensitivity or allergy.

In the same year, Goodale showed that if an individual who was sensitized to a given proteid was exposed to a soluble solution of this proteid in sufficient concentration, by a scratch on the skin, there would be a reaction. He described the classic skin prick test (wheal and flare reaction). Goodale felt that the occurrence of this skin reaction was an indication of sensitization to that proteid; he carefully described the different degrees of intensity of the skin reactions, noticing that they were not always proportional to the intensity of the nasal or other symptoms.

In 1921, Prausnitz and Kustner first demonstrated passive transfer of local sensitivity (P–K reaction) by injecting the serum of a fish-sensitive person into the skin of a normal individual. This subsequently elicited a specific positive skin test for fish at that site. The P–K reaction appeared to offer a safe alternative method for allergy diagnosis. At that time, as is still the case today, skin testing had certain inherent difficulties and dangers.

In describing the P–K reaction in an article published in 1925, Walzer and Kramer stated: "In testing the skin for conditions of atopic hypersensitiveness, the clinician, whether he employs the scratch or intradermal method, is often confronted with numerous difficulties. He is handicapped in the testing of infants and small children, where the patient's cooperation is usually lacking, and the danger of constitutional reactions is always imminent. At times, an irritable skin, or the presence of dermatographia, eczyma, or erythema seriously interferes with the performance and interpretation of the tests."

In 1923, Coca and Grove made use of the P–K reaction in an exhaustive study of the properties of the transferred factor which they termed "Atopic Reagin."

It would take another 50 years, until 1966, for the Ishizakas in the United States, and Benich and Johansson in Sweden, to identify Atopic Reagin as an immunoglobulin. In 1968, the World Health Organization designated the name immunoglobulin E (IgE) to this antibody responsible for mediating hypersensitivity allergic reactions.

In 1967, Wide, Bennich, and Johansson developed the first assay for the measurement of IgE, the Radio-allergosorbent Test (RAST test, as it is now universally called). Since that time, various modifications of the assay have occurred, utilizing the latest technologies and advances in enzyme measurement, monoclonal antibody synthesis, and computerized data reduction, all to be discussed in detail in this manual.

Unfortunately, in the United States, even after 25 years, much of this new knowledge has been denied to patients. Skin testing techniques, which are essentially unchanged from those first described by Goodale in 1916, predominate among conventional allergists. Whether this is due in part to tradition, to economics, or to turf protection, allergists have been loath to embrace *in vitro* testing in the routine evaluation of their allergy patients, despite the fact that today, *in vitro* assays have been shown to be efficacious and cost effective, and are now being used as primary methods of allergy diagnosis in almost every country outside the United States.

It is to the credit of otolaryngic allergists that *in vitro* allergy testing has been readily embraced as part of their allergy management, thus ensuring their patients the very best and safest method that modern medicine has to offer in allergy diagnosis.

I hope this manual will serve to educate and enlighten not only otolaryngologists, but others involved with the management of allergic patients, such as family physicians, internists, pediatricians, pulmonologists, dermatologists, and even conventional allergists.

Ivor A. Emanuel, M.D.

Immunology of IgE Mediated Disease

RICHARD G. FADAL, M.D.

IgE Mediated Hypersensitivity Reactions

The expansion of knowledge about the immunobiologic responses of allergy has followed several pathways. Three of these processes stand in the forefront and will be the focal points of this chapter: the immediate reaction, the late reaction, and the role of cytokines in allergy. Allergists have characteristically focused on immediate events: the short-lived reaction. Late reactions have been poorly understood until recently but are now known to be characterized by inflammation, cellular infiltration, and tissue destructive processes. Recently, the role of several cytokines has been intimately associated with various aspects of atopy, including the regulation of immunoglobulin E (IgE) synthesis, eosinophilia, mast-cell proliferation, and inflammation. These processes will be presented under three separate headings.

The Immediate Allergic Reaction

The allergic state requires two phases before an immediate allergic reaction is possible: a sensitizing step and a subsequent challenge.[1,2]

THE SENSITIZATION PHASE

This process begins when the immune system of a genetically predisposed individual encounters a protein antigen with the appropriate molecular configuration to serve as an allergen.[2] Initially, the foreign substance enters the bloodstream directly (injection) or indirectly, via the respiratory mucosa (pollen) or gastrointestinal tract (food).[2] At this point, interaction with other cells of the immune system must occur for sensitization to be completed.[3] Collaboration between B cells and T cells is essential for induction of antibody response to most protein antigens.[4] Interaction of macrophages or other antigen processing cells (endothelial cells, synovial cells, astrocytes, osteoclasts, and others) with the allergen is an essential initial step.[2] The antigen-presenting macrophage, which is the principal but not exclusive antigen-presenting cell, responds to antigen by secreting a soluble factor and macrophage product, interleukin 1 (IL-1).

IL-1 is a lymphocyte-activating factor that stimulates precursor helper T cells to differentiate into mature helper T cells. Mature helper cells secrete a second soluble factor, interleukin 2 (IL-2). IL-2, a helper T cell product, is a potent immune stimulator capable of promoting clonal expansion of helper T cells and stimulating differentiation of B cells into antibody-secreting plasma cells. IL-2 ensures that only T cells specific for the antigen inciting the immune response will become activated. (The role of IL-4 is pivotal and will be discussed later.) Whatever the mechanism, IgE antibody synthesis is a T-cell dependent immune process.[5,6] Once this process is complete, each plasma cell elaborates antibodies of a single chemical composition, single immunoglobulin class, single specificity, and single sequence of amino acid.[7] The IgE antibody molecules produced are specific and combine through their Fab fragment only with the antigen that stimulated their synthesis. Immunoglobulins of other isotypic specificities are produced but are of no consequence in allergic sensitization.[4]

Once synthesis is complete, IgE antibodies traverse two pathways. The first is diffusion into adjacent lymphoid tissues where encounters with mast cells occur. The IgE antibodies bind to specific IgE Fc receptors on tissue mast cells.[4] The second pathway finds IgE antibodies transported into the blood serum. (Similar binding occurs to specific IgE Fc receptors on blood basophilic leukocytes.[4]) IgE antibody is also circulated to distant lymphoid tissues where additional mast cells are encountered and binding occurs. Through this latter pathway IgE antibodies are synthesized in respiratory or gastrointestinal lymphoid tissue and consequentially bind to mast cells in the skin and other organs. The minimum concentrations of IgE antibodies required for sensitizing normal human skin for a positive PK reaction is 0.2–0.3 ng/ml.[3,4]

In tissue, high-affinity bound IgE is detected on mast cells but not on other cells.[4] However, low-affinity receptors on the surface membrane of macrophages, eosinophils and other cells may bind IgE and contribute to allergen-

IgE induced inflammation. The binding of IgE with mast cells is reversible; however, the affinity of IgE for mast cells and basophils is quite high under physiologic conditions.[4,8] The equilibrium constant of binding between IgE and high-affinity cell receptors is 10^{-9}M.[4,8] The high affinity of IgE for receptors on target cells (mast cells and basophils) explains why a minute dose of IgE antibody can sensitize the cells and why sensitization is persistent.[4] The set of events just discussed is known as the sensitization phase and occurs with the initial encounter and interaction with a foreign allergen.[3]

THE CHALLENGE PHASE

The challenge phase of the allergic state begins with a second exposure and interaction of sensitized host cells with an allergen.[2] A divalent antigen bridges two adjacent, cell-bound IgE molecules of identical specificity and brings the two receptor molecules into close proximity.[9-11] This local disturbance of membrane structures or interaction between adjacent receptor molecules activates membrane-associated enzymes. Enzymes then trigger the cell to release vasoactive amines and other pharmacologically active substances responsible for the clinical manifestations of IgE-mediated immediate hypersensitivity.[12,13]

The active biological complex in IgE-mediated reactions consists of two molecules of IgE, one antigen molecule, and one mediator-containing cell.[14] Evidence indicates that a single active biological complex can secrete detectable quantities of histamine and other inflammatory mediators.[14] In atopic patients, it is unusual for all mediator-cell receptor sites to be occupied by IgE molecules. However, full saturation of about 80,000 to 90,000 receptor sites with IgE can be accomplished under experimental conditions.[4] The binding of IgE antibody to mediator cell receptors is directly related to serum IgE concentration.[9] The higher the serum level of IgE, the greater the binding of IgE to mast cells and basophils and the greater the patient's sensitivity.[9] The greater the patient's sensitivity, the less antigen required to initiate an allergic response.[9] It is axiomatic that the number and nature of cell-bound IgE antibody molecules determines the sensitivity of the cells to an antigen.[4,9,14]

Cross-linking of cell-bound IgE results in complex, enzyme-associated biochemical events. These culminate in a decline of intracellular cyclic adenosine monophosphate (cAMP) and the facilitation of degranulation of mast cells with release of granules containing histamine and other preformed mediators into the microenvironment.[12,13,15] Degranulation is the series of biochemical events involved in the immediate hypersensitivity response. We now call this the activation-secretion response. The result of the activation-secretion response is allergic inflammation. The tissue responds with vasodilation, smooth muscle contraction, increased postcapillary edema, mucous gland secretion, platelet activation, eosinophilic and neutrophilic accumulation, proteolytic tissue damage, inflammatory cell accumulation, and other postinflammatory activities.[2,12,13]

THE ACTIVATION-SECRETION RESPONSE

Mast-cell-membrane IgE Fc receptors are linked to adenylate cyclase activated by the antigen–IgE antibody combination.[12] The substrate for adenylate cyclase is adenosine triphosphate (ATP). ATP is reduced to adenosine monophosphate (AMP), with the resultant activation of a cyclic AMP-dependent protein kinase.[12] All of this leads to a series of biochemical events, still incompletely understood, but associated with intracellular microtubular assembly, which causes the cytoplasmic granules of the mast cell to migrate to the cell surface and fuse with each other and then with the cell membrane.[12] This exocytosis leads to extrusion of the granules to the external microenvironment of the cell.[12] That sequence provides the first of the soluble mediators of immediate hypersensitivity, histamine.[12]

Mast-cell-membrane structures involved in the initial steps of the activation–secretion response include IgE receptors linked to a transmembrane coupling protein and the catalytic subunit of adenylate cyclase.[12] When two IgE molecules are bridged by an antigen, the coupling protein unit activates adenylate cyclase. Cytoplasmic ATP is then used to produce cAMP, which recruits a cytoplasmic, cAMP-dependent protein kinase. Next, cAMP binds to the two regulatory units of the inactive kinase, liberating a catalytic unit that phosphorylates another protein, using additional ATP in the process.[12] The consumption of cAMP facilitates intracellular microtubular assembly, a calcium-dependent reaction, that enhances release of inflammatory mediators.

For many years it was presumed that histamine was the exclusive mediator of the immediate hypersensitivity response.[12,16,17] However, additional mediators were identified as residing with histamine in the secretory granule and arising de novo from membrane fatty acids.[12]

The Late-Phase Reaction and Dual Responses

It is possible to relate the IgE-dependent release of preformed secretory granule-contained mediators and cell-membrane-derived lipid mediators from mast cell and other cell types to clinical allergic events. An allergic response of the mucous membrane, smooth muscle, or skin comprises an immediate event and, in many cases, a late event. Involvement may be with both primary and secondary mediators (Fig. 1–1).[18,54] Following allergen challenge in a sensitized individual, the secretion–release reaction and the release of newly generated lipid-derived mediators is rapid.[17] The immediate response is likely to include vasopermeability, vasoconstriction, smooth muscle spasm, mucous hypersecretion, or myocardial depression, depending on the target tissue of the allergic reaction.[17] This immediate reaction is caused by the combined actions of histamine, platelet-activating factor (PAF), leukotriene C (LTC), and prostaglandin D_2 (PGD_2). Simultaneously, histamine and PGD_2, acting as chemokinetic factors, will attract neutrophils and

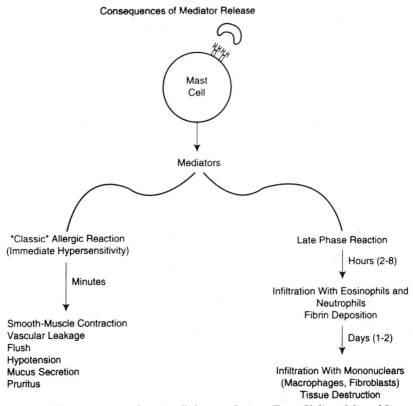

Figure 1–1. Consequences of mast cell degranulation. (From Kaliner M, and Lemanske R, page 2810, Figure 3–6; American Association of Immunologists. Reprinted by permission.)[54]

eosinophils to the area of inflammation as a late event.[17] Hours after the initial IgE-dependent event and after the immediate effector response, these inflammatory cells will infiltrate the reaction site of the target tissues. The cells may become activated by immune complexes of antigen and antibody or by other postinflammatory mechanisms in the mediator-rich, inflammatory-cell-laden, amplification molecule-enhanced microenvironment. Cells could also generate more peptidolipid leukotrienes, PAF-, C3a-, and C5a-derived anaphylatoxins and cause a stronger late-phase response.[17,19]

Allergists have characteristically focused on immediate events, the short-lived reactions.[20] Delayed or late-phase reactions were poorly understood.[20] The possibilities of circulating allergens with delayed absorption or of an inflammatory reaction unrelated to the IgE-dependent mechanism clouded the issue. Focus is now on the acute allergic reaction or immediate hypersensitivity reaction as the first phase of a multisequence reaction that persists for one or two days.[20] Late-phase reactions are characterized by inflammation and infiltration by eosinophils and neutrophils and fibrin deposition. This late-phase inflammatory reaction, which can be a destructive process, follows immediate hypersensitivity responses by two to eight hours and persists for 24 to 48 hours or longer. The intensity of the late-phase reaction usually parallels the intensity of the immediate reaction. It is necessary to understand that the dual allergic reaction and the initiating event in allergic diseases evokes biochemical events more complex than those leading to the release of preformed mast cell secretory granule mediators. The functional efficacy of the newly generated lipid mediators is significant for allergic pathology. The latter compounds in the allergic process should, therefore, be the subject of efforts for future therapeutic intervention.[17]

Though the late-phase reaction is still under investigation, several important aspects of this reaction have been clarified. Approximately 50% (19–84%) of immediate hypersensitivity reactions will be followed by a late response. The late response is more likely to occur if the patient is highly sensitive to the relevant allergen or exposure is high or prolonged. The lung is a preferred target tissue, particularly small airways, but late-phase reactions have been documented in the nose as well. This reaction usually follows the immediate allergic response by two to eight hours and is characterized by infiltration of inflammatory cells resulting in tissue induration, mucus impaction, and tissue destruction. The late-phase reaction is indolent and prolonged for several days and leaves the affected airways hyperreactive for several weeks. Pharmacological agents usually effective for immediate reactions are useless for the late reaction. Corticosteroids are therapeutic, whereas cromolyn and immunotherapy are prophylactic. As for the immediate allergic reaction, avoidance, when practical, is the management procedure of choice. A sequence of reoccurring late reactions superimposed one upon the other can lead to chronic disease and irreversible tissue destruction. Hence, the late-phase reaction is a major contributor to the morbidity associated with allergic diseases.

Nonimmune Mast-Cell Degranulation

The interaction of allergens and specific IgE antibodies on the surface of tissue mast cells or blood basophils is a requirement for a specific immune, IgE-dependent degranulation to occur. It is not an essential step for de novo degranulation of mediator cells. Degranulation and secretion of pharmacoactive mediators can be induced by initiating events besides allergen-IgE interactions (Fig. 1–2).[9] These nonimmune, nonatopic stimuli can cause reactions that simulate allergy and may be clinically indistinguishable because a common pathway of inflammation is employed.[3] Such phenomena are often referred to as "pseudoallergic" or anaphylactoid reactions.[21] It is apparent that in conditions where no allergen can be found as the cause of "apparently" allergic reactions, this mechanism is operative. These "pseudo-

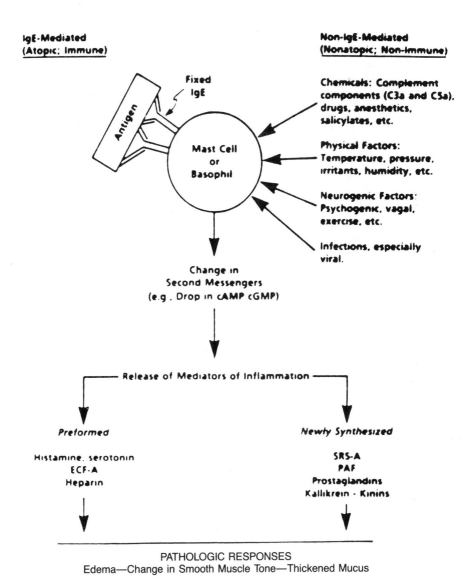

TRIGGERS FOR "ALLERGIC" REACTIONS

IgE-Mediated
(Atopic; Immune)

Non-IgE-Mediated
(Nonatopic; Non-Immune)

Fixed
IgE

Antigen

Mast Cell
or
Basophil

Chemicals: Complement
components (C3a and C5a),
drugs, anesthetics,
salicylates, etc.

Physical Factors:
Temperature, pressure,
irritants, humidity, etc.

Neurogenic Factors:
Psychogenic, vagal,
exercise, etc.

Infections, especially
viral.

Change in
Second Messengers
(e.g., Drop in cAMP cGMP)

———— Release of Mediators of Inflammation ————

Preformed

Histamine, serotonin
ECF-A
Heparin

Newly Synthesized

SRS-A
PAF
Prostaglandins
Kallikrein - Kinins

PATHOLOGIC RESPONSES
Edema—Change in Smooth Muscle Tone—Thickened Mucus

Figure 1–2.   Triggers for allergic reactions. (From Fadal RG, Nalebuff DJ, and Ali M, page 669, Figure 9. Reprinted with permission.)[9]

allergies" include upper and lower airway, gastrointestinal, and cutaneous conditions. Clinically and experimentally, a number of agents have been identified that can stimulate mast cell and basophil secretion.[21] These agents act directly on the mast cell or basophil membrane to bring about the same biochemical alterations and release of mediators that take place in IgE-dependent reactions. Some of the nonimmune stimulators are endogenous products (complement components, acetylcholine, prostaglandins, and hormones). Others are extrinsic chemicals or drugs (anesthetics, radioiodinated contrast media, salicylates, bile salts, antibiotics, sulfonamides). Other nonatopic triggering events include weather changes, airborne irritants, pollution, exercise, stress, and respiratory infections (Table 1–1).[20]

Experimentally, mast cell or basophil secretion can be stimulated by anaphylatoxins (C3a and C5a), calcium ionophores, concanavalin A and other lectins, anti-IgE and antilight chain sera, protein A, formylmethionyl peptides, compound 48/80, opiates (morphine, codeine, meperidine), antibiotics (polymyxin), other drugs (thiamine, d-tubocurarine, stilbamidine, dextran, and other histamine-releasing drugs), certain foods containing or releasing histamine, radiographic contrast media, lymphocytes, and other cell products (cytokines).

A variety of agents and mechanisms may be responsible for release of pharmacological mediators. Some patients may have simultaneous IgE-dependent and IgE-independent mechanisms. The interpretation of the co-existence of such mechanisms is a demanding exercise in differential diagnosis. The precise demonstration of the presence and participation of specific IgE antibodies in such patients is critical.

Table 1–1   **Triggers of Mediator Release**

NONIMMUNE–NONATOPIC TRIGGERS		
Endogenous	*Exogenous*	*Nonspecific Triggers*
Acetylcholine	Anesthestics	Weather changes
Complement components	Radioiodinated contrast	Respiratory infections
Prostaglandins	media	Exercise
Estrogens	Salicylates	Air pollution
	Antibiotics	Anxiety
		Stress

Various nonimmune agents may directly or indirectly perturb mast cells. Agents which either decrease cAMP or increase cGMP favor mediator release. Cholinergic and a-adrenergic autonomic nervous system stimulation through the vagus nerve produces a rise in cGMP, resulting in increased mediator release. B-Adrenergic stimulation through the adenylate cyclase receptor raises intracellular cAMP levels and inhibits mediator release. Many nonspecific triggers are associated with cholinergic autonomic stimulation, producing an increase of intracellular cGMP and associated release of mediators. (From Fadal, RG, Nalebuff, DJ, and Ali, M. With permission.)[9]

The Cyclic Nucleotide and Autonomic Systems

Whatever the precise mechanisms may be, the activation of mast cells and basophils is modulated by their intracellular cAMP concentration.[3,22] Normally a balance exists between intracellular levels of cAMP and those of cyclic guanine monophosphate (cGMP), with the effects of cAMP predominating.[3,22] Elevated levels of cAMP lead to decreased secretion of inflammatory mediators. Elevated cGMP leads to increased mediator secretion.[3,22] Additionally, an imbalance of the autonomic nervous system may be superimposed on and coexist with cyclic nucleotide and/or immunologic imbalance.[22] The interaction of these three separate but interwoven systems leads to a heterogeneity of potential pathologic mechanisms.[20]

The autonomic nervous system is composed of the parasympathetic (cholinergic) and the sympathetic (adrenergic) systems.[22] These systems exert opposing effects on mediator cells, various tissues, and organs (Fig. 1–3).[3] A balance between these systems maintains homeostatic control over mediator cells, target cells, tissues, or organs. In the mast cell and basophil, the release of mediators can be modulated by adrenergic and cholinergic agonists. Similarly, in target tissues, such as bronchial smooth muscle, the tone of the muscles can be determined by the balance between adrenergic or cholinergic activity.[22]

Autonomic nervous system responses are exerted through the cyclic nucleotide system. Stimulation of the parasympathetic cholinergic system through the vagus nerve leads to the production of acetylcholine, activation of cGMP, and mediator release.[22] Stimulation of the sympathetic adrenergic system has

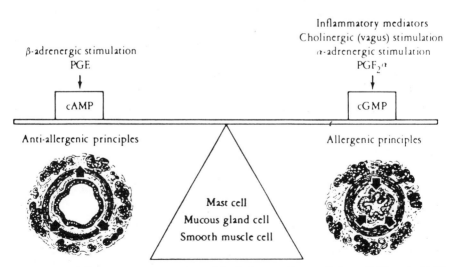

Figure 1–3. Schematic representation of the balance of intracellular cAMP and cGMP and various factors that affect this balance. (From Bellanti J, page 369, Figure 20–17. Reprinted with permission.)[22]

two possible effects. First, stimulation of the alpha receptors leads to decreased levels of intracellular cAMP and enhanced mediator release. Second, stimulation of the beta receptors leads to elevated cAMP and inhibition of mediator release.[22] The degradation of both cAMP and cGMP is accomplished through the enzymatic action of phosphodiesterase.[22]

Acetylcholine acts as the first messenger for the parasympathetic system, while catecholamines act as the first messengers for the sympathetic cyclic nucleotide system.[3,22] The alpha and beta receptors of the sympathetic nervous system are stimulated differently by various endogenous agonists. Norepinephrine, released at the adrenergic nerve terminal, has an alpha effect.[22] Epinephrine, secreted by the adrenal medulla, exerts a predominate beta effect. Exogenous adrenergic agonists specific for the beta receptor exist. Two types of beta receptors, beta 1 and beta 2, have a variable distribution in tissues.[22] The beta 1 receptor exists in cardiac tissue; the beta 2 receptor in pulmonary tissue (Table 1–2). Recent development of specific beta 2 agonists has improved the therapeutics for bronchoconstrictive disorders.

The balance within both mediator cells and target cells is influenced by autonomic activity, the levels of cAMP and cGMP, and a variety of other reactants, such as histamine, beta-adrenergic compounds, PGE, PCF2, and acetylcholine.[21,22] Accordingly, the agents that affect cellular cyclic nucleotide levels or autonomic activity have a predictable effect on mediator release. cAMP levels increase and mediator release decreases after *in vivo* or *in vitro* exposure to theophylline (which inhibits cAMP degradation) or agents that stimulate adenylate cyclase to enhance cAMP production from ATP.[22] The latter include a variety of beta-adrenergic compounds, prostaglandins of the E series, and histamines acting through H2 receptors on mediator cells. Conversely, stimulation of mediator release occurs through the enhanced production of cGMP from GTP by guanylate cyclase activation by acetylcholine (vagal stimulation), prostaglandins of the F series, or histamine through H1 receptors.[21] Histamine can also stimulate vagal irritant receptors and promote increased levels of cGMP by acetylcholine.

Mediator release is energy dependent and requires glycolytic sources as well as calcium ions.[21] Increased levels of cGMP or deuterium oxide facilitate microtubule aggregation and promote the secretory phase of mediator re-

Table 1–2   Beta Receptor Subtypes

SUBTYPE	EFFECTS	AGONISTS
Beta-1	Cardiac inotropic and chronotropic responses	Isoproterenol
Beta-2	Bronchial, vascular, and uterine smooth muscle relaxation	Isoproterenol Epinephrine Albutarol Isoetharine Epinephrine
	Glycogenolysis	

lease.[21] Raised levels of cAMP or colchicine promote microtubular dissociation and inhibit the secretory phase of mediator release.[21]

The target tissues of the allergic inflammatory response are also influenced by the relative balance of the cyclic nucleotides. Raised levels of cAMP modulate the physiological state of the tissues and lead to relaxation of smooth muscles, vasoconstriction, and decreased mucous gland activity. Decreased levels of cAMP have the opposite effect.[22] The released mediators also have an effect on the target tissue, acting through receptors on the surface of target cells. The mediators can exert their effects secondarily by causing subepithelial irritant receptors to exert a cholinergic effect on the target cells. In all aspects of the cyclic nucleotide system, the effects of cGMP appear to be opposite those of cAMP.[22]

The genetic defect associated with a dysfunction or deficiency of T-cell regulatory substances, which leads to the persistent production of IgE antibodies, is related to the partial beta-adrenergic blockade, with an enhanced propensity for mediator release and an autonomic nervous system imbalance. This leads to hypersensitivity of the end organ. In its total aspect, the atopic state is characterized by abnormalities of the immune system through both its humoral- and cell-mediated arms, as well as the cyclic nucleotide system, the autonomic nervous system, cytokines, and other biological response mediators.

Cytokines and Allergy

Immunologic response to a foreign antigen involves participation of numerous cell types and their associated secreted products and results in an antigen-specific effector response. A given antigen may produce antibody mediated immunity, cell mediated immunity, or, alternatively, immunologic tolerance.[23] A different effector response to a particular antigen may be produced in different individuals. Cytokines, which are newly synthesized cell-secreted peptides that regulate immune responses, are critically important in determining the form an immune response takes.[23] In contrast to antibody and T- lymphocyte receptors, cytokines are not antigen specific but may be antigen stimulated.[23–25]

Cytokines modulate the function of virtually all cell types and are themselves produced by many different types of cells.[23–25] Cytokines were originally thought to be lymphocyte or monocyte derived and were erroneously referred to as "lymphokines" or "monokines." It is now established that these immunoactive peptides may be produced by virtually any cell and are more appropriately termed "cytokines."[23]

There are four main groups of cytokines based on their biological functions (Table 1–3).[23–25] The interferons (IFN) were the first of these biological response modifiers to be identified from their potent antiviral activities.[26] Colony-stimulating factors (CSF) are peptides that induce maturation of bone

Table 1–3   Cytokines

INTERFERONS	CSF	TNF	INTERLEUKINS
IFN-α	IL-3	TNF-α	IL1-10
IFN-β	IL-5	TNF-β	MIPs
IFN-γ	GM-CSF		
	G-CSF		
	M-CSF		

IFN: interferon, CSF: colony stimulating factor, IL: interleukin, GM: granulocyte/macrophage, G: granulocyte, M: macrophage, TNF: tumor necrosis factor, MIP: macrophage inflammatory peptide. (From Borish, L, page 2, Table 1. Reprinted with permission.)[23]

marrow precursor cells into circulating cells.[23,24,27,28] Tumor necrosis factors (TNF) have the capacity to destroy cancerous tumor cells by inducing hemorrhagic necrosis.[23,24,29,30] The interleukins (IL) are the largest, the most heterogeneous, and the most important group of cytokines. Their name is derived from their capacity to deliver "inter-leukocyte" signals. ILs mediate interactions between cells of the immune system and between other cell types. These powerful cytokines are completely capable of mobilizing the entire organism in the immune response (Table 1–4).[23,24]

The excessive production of IgE antibodies, the hallmark of atopic allergy,

Table 1–4   Cytokines and Allergy

	CYTOKINE	ACTIVITY
IgE regulation	IL-4	IgE isotype switch
	IL-2, IL-5, IL-6	Synergizes with IL-4
	IFN-γ	Inhibits IL-4
	IL-10	Inhibits IFN-γ (enhances IgE production)
Eosinophilia	IL-3, IL-5, GM-CSF	Eosinophilopoietins
Mast cell development and activation	IL-3, IL-9, IL-10	Mast cell growth factor
	Hematopoietic stem cell factor	
	CTAP-III	Histamine-releasing factor
Inflammation	IFN-γ, GM-CSF, G-CSF, TNFs, IL-1, IL-4, IL-6, IL-8	Neutrophil-activating factors
	GM-CSF, TNFs, IL-1, IL-3, IL-5	Eosinophil-activating factors
	IFN-γ, GM-SCF, M-CSF, TNFs, IL-1, IL-2, IL-3, IL-4	Macrophage-activating factors

IL: interleukin, CSF: colony-stimulating factor, IFN: interferon, TNF: tumor necrosis factor, CTAP: connective tissue-activating peptide, G: granulocyte, M: macrophage. (From Borish, L, page 6, Table 5. Reprinted with permission.)[23]

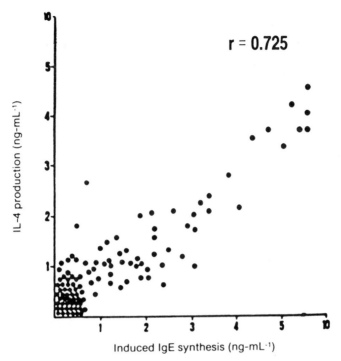

Figure 1–4.   The ability of human T-cell clones to induce IgE synthesis corresponds to their ability to produce IL-4. Each clone (1×10^6 blasts/mL) was stimulated for 24 hours with PHA (1 μg/mL), and the cell-free supernatant was assayed for IL-4 by ELISA. T-cell blasts from each clone were also cultured for 10 days with B cells from two different donors, and supernatants from these cultures were assayed for their IgE content by RIA. Mean values from duplicate IL-4 determinations are plotted against mean values of duplicate IgE determinations. (From Borish L, page 6, Figure 3. Reprinted with permission.)[23]

is the function of the opposing actions of IL-4 and IFN-g.[23,31–33] IL-4 directly induces the synthesis of IgE antibodies by B lymphocytes (Fig. 1–4).[23,31–33] While IL-4 is necessary for IgE production, it is not sufficient. The secretion of IgE by B cells requires additional T-cell-derived signals.[34] Additionally, IL-2, IL-5, and IL-6 synergize with IL-4 to increase secretion of IgE. The most important function of IL-4 for atopy is the ability of IL-4 to stimulate the immunoglobulin isotype switch from IgM to IgE.[23,33]

IFN-g specifically inhibits the IL-4 mediated isotype switch to IgE, and the capacity of T-cell clones to support the IgE synthesis is inversely proportional to IFN-g production (Fig. 1–5).[23,33] The output of IgE antibodies in atopy represents a combination of adequate stimulation by IL-4 and the relative absence of IFN-g production.[23,34,35] Studies have shown that allergen-specific T-cell clones harvested from atopic subjects are more likely to produce IL-4 and not IFN-γ than are similar T-cell clones obtained from nonatopic individ-

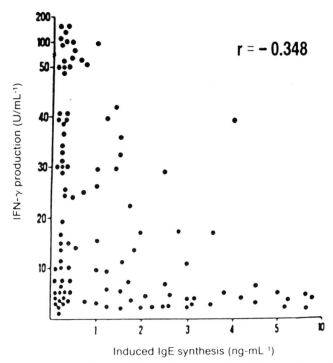

Figure 1–5.   The ability of human T-cell clones to induce IgE synthesis is inversely proportional to their ability to produce IFN-γ. Each clone was used to stimulate B cells from two different donors, as described for Figure 4. IgE and IFN-γ quantifications were performed by RIA. IFN-γ determinations are plotted against mean IgE values. (From Borish, L, page 7, Figure 4. Reprinted with permission.)[23]

uals.[36] The most recently discovered interleukin (IL-10) inhibits IFN-g production by T cells and potentiates IgE synthesis.[37,38]

OTHER ASPECTS OF CYTOKINES IN ALLERGY

Eosinophils. In addition to excessive IgE antibody production, another characteristic feature of atopy is the presence of increased numbers of circulating and tissue localized eosinophils. Eosinophilia is a T-cell mediated response, as evidenced by its absence in T-cell-depleted animals.[39,40] IL-5 is the most important eosinophilopoitin and eosinophil-activating factor.[23] IL-5 is essential for the development of eosinophilia, but IL-3 and granulocyte/macrophage colony stimulating factor (GM-CSF) may also contribute.[23] The ability to someday inhibit IL-5 may prevent eosinophil-mediated tissue damage.

Mast cells. Mast-cell proliferation, like excessive IgE production and eosinophilia, is characteristic of allergic diseases and is also a T-cell dependent process.[23,40–42] The cytokines IL-3, IL-9, and IL-10 have been shown to stimulate proliferation of mast cells. Significantly, IL-3, IL-8 and GM-CSF are capable of inducing histamine release from mast cells.[23] It has recently been shown that mast cells may produce cytokines. Mast cell proliferation induced by IL-3 may be inhibited by GM-CSF.

Inflammation. The classical atopic diseases, allergic rhinitis, asthma, and atopic eczema, are characterized by inflammation and damage to resident tissue.[23,24] A number of allergic mediators are capable of recruitment and activation of eosinophils and neutrophils. Compared with histamine, leukotrienes, prostaglandins, platelet activating factor, and other preformed or generated mediators, cytokines are particularly potent, stable, and longlasting inflammatory mediators. It appears that all classes of cytokines may participate in the induction of allergen-induced inflammation.[23,24] Recent evidence indicates that cytokine secretion may be an essential component for the development of allergic inflammation.[23,43]

IgE regulation. T cells do not necessarily produce all of their cytokines at the time of activation.[23] T-helper cell (TH) have been identified and contain a distinct repertoire of cytokines (Table 1–5, Figure 1–6).[23] In addition to producing distinct classes of cytokines, TH_1 and TH_2 cells are mutually inhibitory. In animal experiments, TH_1 cells promoted cell mediated immunity, whereas TH_2 cells induced B-cell maturation and supported antibody-dependent immunity.[23,45-47] This T-helper cell dichotomy is less distinct in humans. Nevertheless, the observation that the capacity of a given T-cell clone to stimulate IgE synthesis is directly proportional to the amount of IL-4 (TH_2 cells) it produces and inversely proportional to the amount of IFN-γ (TH_1 cells) produced supports the concept that human TH_2 cells may be essential in mediating allergic diseases.[23,45-49]

The Future. In addition to producing cytokines, the immune system has the capacity to synthesize specific cytokine antagonists. Inhibitors of IL-1, IL-8, and TNFs have recently been identified.[23,50-53] Through the administration of cytokines or cytokine inhibitors, it is possible to manipulate the nature of the immune response.[23] The relevance to allergy is profound, as there is irrefutable evidence that the basis for the development of allergic diseases is medi-

Table 1–5 Helper Subtypes

Th1	Th2	BOTH
IFN-γ	IL-4	GM-CSF
IL-2	IL-5	IL-3
TNF-β	IL-6	
	IL-10	

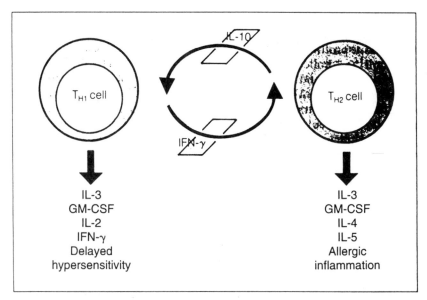

Figure 1–6. Two distinct populations of T-cells each secrete different profiles of cytokines; those from TH_1 lead to delayed hypersensitivity, whereas those from TH_2 lead to allergic inflammation. (GM-CSF, granulocyte-macrophage colony-stimulating factor; IL, interleukin; IFN-γ, interferon-γ). (From Lamanske RF Jr, page S12, Figure 2. Reprinted with permission.)[44]

Table 1–6   Some of the Immunomolecular Biological Response Substances Under Investigation

FUNCTION	DESCRIPTION
CGRP	Calcitonin gene-related peptide
CPR	Gastrin-releasing peptide
CTAP	Connective tissue-activating peptide
ELAM-1	Endothelial leukocyte adhesion molecule
FceRI	High affinity IgE receptor
FceRII	Low affinity IgE receptor (CD23)
HRF	Histamine releasing factors
ICAM-1	Intercellular adhesion molecule-1
LFA	Lymphocyte function-associated antigen
MIP	Macrophage inflammatory protein
NKA	Neurokinnin A
PBP	Platelet basic protein
SP	Substance P
VIP	Vasoactive intestinal peptide

Table 1–7   **Mast Cell-Derived Mediators***

Preformed mediators rapidly released under physiological conditions:
    Histamine
    Eosinophil and neutrophil chemotactic factors
    Kininogenase
    Tumor necrosis factor a
    Interleukin 6
    Endothelin-1
    Arylsulfatase A
    Exoglycosidases (B-hexosaminidase, B-D-galactosidase, B-glucuronidase)

Mediators formed during the degranulation process:
    Superoxide and other reactive oxygen species
    Leukotrienes C4, D4, E4 (previously known as SRS-A)
    PGD2, hydroxyeicosatetaraenoic acids, HHT
    Prostaglandin-generating factor of anaphylaxis
    Adenosine
    Bradykinin
    Platelet-activating factor

Mediators closely associated with the granule:
    Heparin, chondroitin sulfate E
    Tryptase
    Chymase
    Cathepsin G
    Carboxypeptidase
    Peroxidase
    Arylsulfatase B
    Inflammatory factors
    Superoxide dismutase

Cytokines generated after activation:
    Interleukins 1, 2, 3, 4, 5, 6
    Granulocyte-macrophage colony-stimulating factor
    Macrophage inflammatory protein 1a and 1B
    Monocyte chemotactic and activating factor
    Tumor necrosis factor a
    TCA-3
    Endothelin-1

*PG: prostaglandin; HHT: hydroxyheptadec-atrinsinoic acid; TCA: T-cell activating gene. (Modified from Costa and Metcalfe. Reprinted with permission.)

ated by the hypersecretion of certain cytokines. The ability to manipulate cytokine activity to reverse or down-regulate the atopic state is a logical and obtainable goal.

While much is known about the immunobiology of atopy, more will be learned of this important and complicated process in the future. Research is unraveling the mysteries of allergic mechanisms. Research in molecular biology has already identified scores of reactants that are implicated in the pathology of atopy (Tables 1–6 and 1–7).[54] Continued investigation into the various and intricate molecular constituents involved in the immunopathology of the atopic response will ultimately lead to improved diagnostic procedures and refined therapeutics.

References

1. Frick OL. Immediate hypersensitivity. In Stites DP, et al, eds. *Basic and Clinical Immunology*. Los Altos, CA: Lange Medical Publications, 1982:250–276.
2. Hamilton RG, Adkinson MF. Clinical laboratory methods in allergy disease. *Lab. Manage.*, December, 1983.
3. Fadal RG, and Nalebuff DJ, eds. *RAST in Clinical Allergy*. Miami: Symposia Specialists, Inc; 1981.
4. Geha RS. Human IgE. *J Allergy Clin Immunol* 1984;74:109–120.
5. Hollman MM. The incidence of allergic disease in a pediatric population. *Conn Med J* 1960;24:632.
6. Ramanarayanan MP. Immunoglobulins and the immune system. *Otolaryngol Clin N Amer* 1985;18:627–647.
7. Ishizaka K, and Ishizaka T. Biology of immunoglobulin E: Molecular basis of reaginic hypersensitivity. *Prog Allergy* 1975;19:60.
8. Ishizaka T, Soto C, and Ishizaka K. Mechanisms of passive sensitization III. Number of IgE molecules and its receptor sites on human basophil granulocytes. *J Immunol* 1973;111:500.
9. Fadal RG, Nalebuff DJ, and Ali M. The allergy problem. In Spencer E, James T, eds. *Allergy Problems: Current Therapy*. Miami: Meded Publishers; 1981.
10. Fadal RG, and Nalebuff DJ. *Tools of the allergist: Old and new*. Continuing Ed. Family Phys. 1979;10:37–61.
11. Ishizaka T. *IgE and mechanisms of IgE-mediated hypersensitivity*. International IgE Symposium Presentation, 1982.
12. Austen KF. The heterogeneity of mast cell populations and products. *Hosp Pract* 1984;19:64–67.
13. Schwartz LB, and Austen KF. Structure and function of the chemical mediators of mast cells. *Prog Allergy* 1984;34:271.
14. Kishimotor T, Hirai Y, Suemura M, et al. Regulation of antibody response in different immunoglobulin classes. Selective suppression of anti-DNP IgE antibody response by preadministration of DNP-coupled mycobacterium. *J Immunol* 1973;111:720.
15. Austen KF. Biologic implications of the structural and functional characteristics of the chemical mediators of immediate-type hypersensitivity. *Harvey Lect* 1979;73:93.
16. Atkins PC. Late onset reactions. *Immunol Allergy Practice* 1984;6:15–19.
17. Lewis RA. The leukotrienes and other mediators of asthma: Newer concepts. *Immunol Allergy Pract* 1984;6:9.
18. Schleimer RP, MacGlashan DW Jr, Peters SP, et al. Inflammatory mediators and mechanisms of release from purified human basophils and mast cells. *J Allergy Clin Immunol* 1984;74: 473–481.
19. Lee CW, Austen KF, Corey EJ, et al. Generation and metabolism of C 6-sulfidopeptide leukotrienes in IgE-dependent reactions: Mast cell heterogeneity. In Piper PJ, ed. *Leukotrienes and Other Lipoxygenase Products*. London: John Wiley and Sons. In press.
20. Fadal RG. The immunobiology and immunopharmacology of the allergic response. *Otolaryngol Clin N Amer* 1985;18:649–676.
21. Settipane GA, ed. Rhinitis. Providence, Rhode Island: The New England and Regional Allergy Proceedings, 1984.
22. Bellanti J. *Immunology III*. Philadelphia: W. B. Saunders Co; 1985.
23. Borish L. Cytokines and allergy. In Middleton E Jr, Reed CE, Ellis EF, Adkinson NF Jr, Yunginger JW, eds. *Allergy, Principles and Practice* (suppl, 3rd ed) St. Louis: C. V. Mosby Co; 1991.
24. Claman HN. The biology of the immune response. *JAMA* 1992;268:2790.
25. Arai K, Lee F, Miyajima A, et al. Cytokines: Coordinators of immune and inflammatory responses. *Ann Rev Biochem* 1990;59:783–836.
26. Isaacs A, Lindermann J. Virus interference. I. The interferon. *Proc R Soc* (Lond.) 1957;147:258.
27. Sieff CA. Hematopoietic growth factors. *J Clin Invest* 1987;79:1549.

28. Cosman D. Colony-stimulating factors *in vivo* and *in vitro*. *Immunol Today* 1988;9:97.
29. Old LJ. Tumor necrosis factor (TNF). *Science* 1985;230:630–632.
30. Beutler B, Cerami A. The biology of cachectin/TNF-A primary mediator of the host response. *Annu Rev Immunol* 1989;7:625.
30. Israel E, and Drazen J. Leukotrienes and asthma: A basic review. *Curr Concepts Allergy Clin Immunol* 1983;16:11–15.
31. Yokata T, Otsuka T, Mosmann T, et al. Isolation and characterization of a human interleukin cDNA clone homologous to mouse BSF-1 that espresses B cell/T cell stimulating activities. *Proc Natl Acad Sci USA* 1986;83:5894.
32. Paul WE, Ohara J. B cell stimulatory factor 1/interleukin 4. *Annu Rev Immunol* 1987;5:429.
33. Coffman RL, Carty J. A T cell activity that enhances polyclonal IgE production and its inhibition by interferon-y. *J Immunol* 1986;136:949.
34. Del Prete GF, Maggi E, Parronchi P, et al. IL-4 is an essential factor for IgE synthesis induced *in vitro* by human T cell clones and their supernatants. *J Immunol* 1988;140:4193.
35. Pene J, Rousset F, Briere F, et al. IgE production by normal human B cells induced by alloreactive T cell clones is mediated by IL-4 and suppressed by IFN-y. *J Immunol* 1988;141:1218.
36. Wierenga EA, Snoek M, deGroot C, et al. Evidence for compartmentalization of functional subsets of CD4+ T lymphokines in atopic patients. *J Immunol* 1990;144:4651.
37. Fioretino DF, Bond MW, Mosmann TR. Two types of mouse T helper cell. IV. Th2 clones secrete a factor that inhibits cytokine production by Th1 clones. *J Exp Med* 1989;170:2081.
38. Moore KW, Vieira P, Fiorentino DF, Trounstine ML, Khan TA, Mosmann TR. Homology of cytokine synthesis inhibitory factor (IL-10) to the Epstein-Barr virus gene BCRF1. *Science* 1990;248:1320.
39. Basten A, Beeson PB. Mechanism of eosinophilia, II. Role of the lymphocytes. *J Exp Med* 1970;131:1288.
40. Katona IM, Urban JF Jr, Finkelman FD. The role of L3T4+ and Lyt-2+ T cells in the IgE response and immunity to Nippostrongylus brasiliensis. *J Immunol* 1988;140:3206.
41. Mayrhofer G. The nature of thymus dependency of mucosal mast cells. II. The effect of thymectomy and of depleting recirculating lymphocytes on the response to Nippostrongylus brasiliensis. *Cell Immunol* 1979;47:312.
42. Ruitenberg EJ, Elgersma A. Absence of intestinal mast cell response in congenitally athymic mice during Trichinella spiralis infections. *Nature* 1976;264:258.
43. Wegner CD, Gundel RH, Reilly P, Haynes N, Letts GL, Rothlein R. Intercellular adhesion molecule-1 (ICAM-1) in the pathogenesis of asthma. *Science* 1990;247:456.
44. Lamanske RF, Jr. Inflammation's role in mild and moderate asthma. *J Respir Dis* (October suppl) 1991:2.
45. Mosmann TR, Cherwinski H, Bond MW, Giedlin MA, Coffman RL. Two types of murine helper T cell clones: 1. Definition according to the profiles of lymphokine activities and secreted proteins. *J Immunol* 1986;136:2348.
46. Killar L, MacDonald G, West J, Woods A, Bottomly K. Cloned, 1a-restricted T cells that do not produce interleukin 4 (IL4)/B cell stimulatory factor 1 (BSF-1) fail to help antigen-specific B cells. *J Immunol* 1987;138:1674.
47. Mosmann TR, Coffman RL. TH1 and TH2 cells: Different patterns of lymphokine secretion lead to different functional properties. *Annu Rev Immunol* 1989;7:145.
48. Gajewski TF, Fitch FW. Antiproliferative effect of 1FN-y in immune regulation. 1. 1FN-y inhibits the proliferation of Th2 but not Th1 murine helper T lymphocyte clones. *J Immunol* 1988;140:4245.
49. Horowitz JB, Kaye J, Conrad PJ, Katz ME, Janeway CA. Autocrine growth inhibitor of a clone line of helper T cells. *Proc Natl Acad Sci USA* 1986;83:1886.
50. Hannum CH, Wilcox CJ, Arend WP, et al. Interleukin-1 receptor antagonist activity of a human interleukin-a inhibitor. *Nature* 1990;343:336.
51. Seckinger P, Isaaz S, Dayer J-M. Purification and biologic characterization of a specific tumor necrosis factor a inhibitor. *J Biol Chem* 1989;264:11966.
52. Lantz M, Gulberg U, Nilsson E, Olsson I. Characterization *in vitro* of a human tumor necrosis factor-binding protein: a soluble form of a tumor necrosis factor receptor. *J Clin Invest* 1990;86:1396.
53. Gimbrone MA Jr, Obin MS, Brock AF, et al. Endothelial interleukin-8: A novel inhibitor of leukocyte-endothelial interactions. *Science* 1989;246:1601.
54. Kaliner M, Lemanske R. Rhinitis and asthma. *JAMA* 1992;268:2810.

The Measurement of Total and Specific IgE Antibody Using In Vitro Assays
A Review of the First Twenty-Five Years

DONALD J. NALEBUFF, M.D.

Background

In 1921 Prausnitz and Kustner[1] injected serum from a fish-sensitive individual into known nonresponders. They noted that the formerly nonreactive recipients of this serum, when appropriately challenged, responded with a positive wheal and flare response. They called this skin-sensitizing serum factor "reagin" and the phenomenon became known as the P–K reaction. The exact nature of this serum factor remained a mystery until 1966 when the Ishizakas[2] isolated a "reagin-rich" immunoglobulin from the serum of an atopic patient. This factor gave a P–K titer of 80,000, or the reciprocal of the highest dilution of serum giving a definite positive reaction. This substance was different from the other known immunoglobulins. Because it appeared to mediate the erythema skin reaction of the allergic response, they called it "gamma E globulin." Simultaneously, Johansson and Bennich[3] isolated an atypical serum protein from a myeloma patient. Minute amounts of this myeloma protein were capable of blocking the P–K reaction. The patient's initials (ND) were adopted as an interim label for this substance. They observed that similar material was present in trace amounts in the serum of patients with hay fever and allergic asthma. Subsequent study established that the "gamma E globulin" and the "N.D. myeloma protein" were the same substance. In 1968, the research finding of these two groups were joined and a new class of immunoglobulin (IgE) was established by the World Health Organization.[4]

Detection of Total IgE

The measurement of total IgE protein was enhanced by the development of two radioimmunoassays using two distinct methods.[5,6] The first method, exemplified by the radioimmunosorbent test (RIST), were inhibition procedures that measure IgE from its capacity to block the reaction between a defined amount of radiolabeled IgE and specific antibodies to IgE; the more IgE there is in a serum sample, the less radioactivity bound to the antibody. In the second method, double-antibody (sandwich) assays such as the paper radioimmunosorbent test (PRIST), there is a direct or positive relationship between IgE concentration and the binding of tracer. While these two diverse techniques give similar responses in the higher concentration range (100 ng and above), there are significant discrepancies in the lower ranges, due either to differences in the sensitivity of the particular test or to false elevations from interfering serum factors. RIST suffers from the presence of the interfering factors, which tend to lead to an overestimate of the amount of IgE in the test sample. This problem is eliminated by the PRIST.

With this new technology, it soon became obvious that presence of IgE was not an abnormal phenomenon limited to allergic patients; it was, in fact, measurable in almost all individuals. We find that the measurement of total serum IgE levels has only limited clinical significance in evaluating allergic patients. The total IgE antibody level can only be correlated with clinical allergy in a general way; that is, patients with higher concentrations of total serum IgE (> 100 units/ml) are usually positive to multiple allergens, and in these patients there is a greater incidence of extremely high levels of specific antibody detected, especially in patients with total IgE levels of 200 units/ml or more. However, in some patients with a total serum IgE level of over 400 units/ml, no positive specific antibody is ever found. Markedly elevated levels have been reported in parasitic diseases and in various immunodeficiency states (Table 2–1). On the other hand, 50% of patients with clinical evidence of allergy and tangible allergen-specific IgE have total IgE levels in ranges usually considered to be within normal limits, and some patients with serum total IgE levels below 50 U/ml have significant specific antibody titres to a limited number of antigens. Patients with total serum IgE levels of 20 U/ml or less, however, rarely have discernible specific IgE levels.

Table 2–1   Elevated Serum Levels of IgE

ALLERGIC DISORDERS	IMMUNOLOGIC DISORDERS OF UNCERTAIN PATHOGENESIS	OTHER CAUSES
Atopic rhinitis and sinusitis	Hyper-IgE and recurrent pyoderma (Job-Buckley syndrome)	IgE myeloma
Atopic asthma		Advanced Hodgkin's disease
Atopic dermatitis and urticaria	Thymic dysplasias and deficiencies	Parasitic infestations
Bronchopulmonary aspergillosis	Wiskott-Aldrich syndrome	
Hypersensivity pneumonitis	Pemphigoid	
Drug and food allergies	Periarteritis nodosa	

Soon after the exact nature of IgE had been determined, Wide, Johansson and Bennich (1967) developed a radioimmunoassay called the Radioallergosorbent Test (RAST) for the detection of specific IgE antibodies in serum.[7] These researchers reported that 27 of 28 patients who could be provoked by an allergen challenge had detectable levels of specific IgE antibody; on the other hand, 21 of 22 nonprovocable patients had no detectable levels. Thus, in 51 patients the test results were correct in 49 determinations. The *in vitro* determination of specific IgE antibody by RAST had a clinical sensitivity, specificity, and overall efficiency of 96%.

RAST was found to be more quantitative than the P-K reaction while obviating the need of a recipient and eliminating the risk of transmitting disease.[8] It was promptly used in the detection of IgE antibodies to pollens, dust components, mold spores, animal danders, and foods.[9–11] Even occupational exposures to industrial chemical substances,[12,13] viruses, and bacteria were found to produce specific IgE antibodies. Early investigators reported a high correlation between RAST scores and the allergic history, the response to allergen challenge, skin end-point titration,[14,15] and the response to pharmacotherapy.[16,17]

Test Performance

The principles of RAST are listed in Table 2–2. In the first stage of the procedure, solid-phase allergens (activated paper discs) are reacted with serum from suspected allergic individuals. IgE antibodies, as well as antibodies of other immunoglobulin classes, react with the allergens present on the solid-phase material and form an antigen–antibody complex. Antibodies not directed against these allergens are washed away. In the second step, the antigen–antibody complexes are reacted with radiolabeled antibodies to

Table 2–2   **Immunologic Principles of the Radioallergosorbent Test**

1. Soluble allergens can be bound to solid-phase supports to create a stable immunosorbent particle, which acquires the antigenicity of the allergen.
2. The passively created immunosorbent (insoluble allergen), on incubation with a test serum, will react with specific antibody to form a solid-phase complex.
3. Anti-human IgE serum raised in another species (rabbit) and radiolabeled with ^{125}I will react with antigenic determinants on the Fc portion of the IgE antibody bound to the allergen-coated immunosorbent.
4. The greater the amount of radioactivity remaining bound to the immune-complex (disc), the more specific IgE present in the serum sample under test. Counts greater than 2× nonspecific background binding are considered to be a positive test.

human IgE. These labeled antibodies react only with the IgE bound to the surface of the solid-phase complex. After a second washing step to remove all unbound labeled anti-IgE, the residual radioactivity is measured in a gamma counter. The amount of radioactivity is directly related to the quantity of specific IgE antibody present in the serum sample.[18] In the original RAST, amounts between two to five times the nonspecific counts obtained with negative controls were scored as positive[7]; those above five times were considered to be strongly positive.

In 1975, Gleich and Yunginger writing about the future and likely role of the RAST in the practice of allergy stated that ". . . the introduction of RAST has been a milestone in the transition of allergy from a practice based on subjective judgments related to history and skin tests to one based on definitive biochemical information derived from the clinical chemistry laboratory."[19] Despite the potential advantages of such testing, only a minority of allergists routinely utilize such measurements. This has occurred, we believe, as the result of the conservative scoring system associated with the first commercially available *in vitro* test for the measurement of specific IgE antibody, the Phadebas RAST (phRAST). This test was about 50% as sensitive as the skin prick test (SPT).

The Phadebas RAST (phRAST)

In the early 1970s, reference laboratories and physicians were provided by Pharmacia Diagnostics with all the reagents necessary to perform their test for the measurement of specific IgE. Included with the basic materials were four reference standards: reference standard A obtained from patients highly allergic to birch pollen, reference standard B (a fivefold dilution of standard A), reference standard C (a fivefold dilution of standard B) and reference standard D (a twofold dilution of standard C). Each of these reference points was assigned PRU units calibrated in-house against a WHO IgE standard, ranging from 50 units for Reference A and one unit for reference D. In the

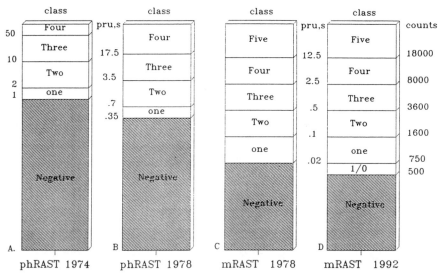

Figure 2–1.   Diagram of the predominant *in vitro* test scoring systems used from 1974–1992. The solid phase used was an activated paper disc.

phRAST scoring system, test sera with bound radioactivity less than one PRU were considered to have non-detectable levels of allergen-specific IgE.

In 1978, however, Deuschl and Johansson described 18 patients with allergic rhinitis who were positive by history, provocation, and the SPT, yet failed to have discernible levels of allergen-specific IgE by the phRAST.[20] They reported that a fivefold dilution of reference standard D still gave binding significantly greater than that of negative controls.[15] By lowering the cut-off point to 0.2 PRU units, they had improved the sensitivity of the test without loss of specificity. 66% of these tests were then recorded as "weakly positive."

In our laboratory,[21] it was observed that a tenfold dilution of reference standard D with human cord serum to 0.1 PRU unit still gave a binding value greater than three times that obtained with negative controls. We suggested that this be adopted as a suitable cutoff for the detection of specific-IgE antibody in the phRAST. In 1979, as a result of these observations and in response to criticisms leveled at its low level of sensitivity, an updated phRAST was introduced. The reference standards had all been diluted only one-third. The reference D cutoff point was now set at 0.35 PRU units; however, this new cut-off level did not solve the problem.

To demonstrate that specific IgE was detectable below this 0.35 PRU unit cutoff point, we performed a series of experiments. An eightfold dilution of the new reference standard D to 0.04 PRU still gave counts equivalent to twice those with the negative control. Moreover, further dilution made it indistinguishable from the nonspecific binding of the negative control. RAST inhibition by preincubation with compatible soluble homologous allergen accomplished the same thing.

The Modified RAST

These observations were applied in the development of the modified RAST (mRAST).[22,23] Several changes were incorporated into the test to optimize sensitivity.[17] First, the initial incubation period was increased from 3 to 24 hours. Lundkvist (1975) had shown that when working with very weak responses this gave the optimal kinetics.[18] Additionally, to guarantee that the allergen disc is kept moist through the entire first incubation period, the volume of the test serum was raised from 50- to 100μ. When we used less test serum, some discs dried out during the overnight incubation. After the second incubation with labeled anti-human IgE and prior to counting the bound radioactivity, we added an extra step. The coated allergen discs were removed from the original polystyrene tubes and before counting were placed into clean tubes. This was done to insure that only radioactivity immunologically bound to the disc was measured. In recent years, with improved reagents and better washing techniques, this step is now super-fluous.

Improved reproducibility of assay results between laboratories is accomplished by using a time or count control; that is, the time used to count each disc matches that required by a WHO standardized 25-unit IgE/ml sample to reach 25,000 counts when tested against an anti-IgE disc and run in parallel to the atopic sera under test. When this was originally done the average nonspecific binding in the mRAST system averaged 500 counts or 2% of that obtained by the 25-unit IgE time control. In the original mRAST system the lower limit of detectable levels of allergen-specific IgE was 750 counts or 1.5 times the mean binding of negative controls. These controls were either human cord serum, serum from nonatopic patients, or serum from highly atopic patients tested against an inappropriate allergen.[18,19]

In the 1992 isotopic mRAST system,[24] 250 counts, or 1% of the 25-unit time control, represent the average nonspecific binding of negative controls tested against different allergen discs. Mean nonspecific binding plus two standard deviations in the mRAST is at 415 counts; thus, 500 counts, or 2% of the time control, is well above the 95% confidence level for the detection of allergen-specific IgE antibody. Scores between 500 and 750 counts are considered to be equivocal; that is, the detected specific IgE antibody may not be clinically relevant. With an enzymatic tracer, the nonspecific binding is somewhat higher, at 375 counts. If enzymatic markers are used, one should keep the cutoff point at 750 counts, or 3% of the time control. Scores above 750 counts are divided into distinct classes, each representing approximately a fivefold increase in the amount of specific IgE antibody present in the sample. mRAST Class 1 (750–1600 counts) is a low level positive score. Class 1 levels are always associated with a positive intradermal skin test reaction, and 70% of affected patients will respond to a nasal or conjunctival challenge. In contrast, mRAST Class 2 scores and above (1600–40,000 counts) represent positive scores, with increasing levels of specific-IgE antibody and degrees of clinical sensitivity, and 95% of patients with these scores respond positively to the appropriate allergen challenge test (Table 2–2).

Over the past 15 years, rigorous peer review of the mRAST has been conducted to evaluate its test qualities. These studies have confirmed that the test is not only sensitive and specific but that results are reproducible and quantitative.[25–29] The most extensive peer review of the mRAST was done by 17 members of the in-vitro committee of the American Academy of Allergy and Immunology.[27] An example of their results with serial dilutions of a serum from a highly sensitive patient to cat epithelium is listed in Table 2–3.

Other *In Vitro* Clones of the RAST

In recent years, numerous additional tests for the measurement of specific IgE have been developed, some are[30–35] listed in Table 2–4. Many provide reagents qualified to perform the mRAST assay as described above. Others have been developed that use enzymatic markers instead of isotopic tags and plastic microtiter plates as the solid-phase support. In these assays, individual

Table 2–3   Modified RAST Scores Obtained with 17 Laboratories

	COUNTS (mRAST CLASS)			
INVESTIGATOR	*Cat X*	*Cat Y*	*Cat Z*	*HSD*
Adkinson	21,693 (5)	6026 (3)	2367 (2)	240 (0)
Baer	19,545 (5)	6365 (3)	3637 (2)	267 (0)
Bernstein	21,953 (5)	7357 (3)	2913 (2)	337 (0)
Curran	22,624 (5)	6265 (3)	3263 (2)	345 (0)
Evans	21,240 (5)	7417 (3)	3014 (2)	346 (0)
Hamburger	21,108 (5)	5136 (3)	2679 (2)	436 (0)
Hoffman	24,722 (5)	7973 (3)	3385 (2)	355 (0)
Krumholz	20,094 (5)	7639 (3)	3015 (2)	266 (0)
Nalebuff	20,498 (5)	5710 (3)	2837 (2)	348 (0)
Perelmutter	21,730 (5)	8483 (3)	2976 (2)	341 (0)
Steinberg	17,644 (5)	8053 (3)	3644 (3)	358 (0)
Targan	20,308 (5)	5923 (3)	2426 (2)	387 (0)
Townley	22,632 (5)	7773 (3)	2889 (2)	441 (0)
Wypych	21,993 (5)	8241 (4)	2672 (2)	298 (0)
Yanari	24,223 (5)	5865 (3)	2875 (2)	312 (0)
Yoo/Tai	21,415 (5)	6775 (3)	2267 (2)	280 (0)
Yunginger	21,963 (5)	7511 (3)	2631 (2)	508 (0)

In 64/68 tests the classes were the same. Similar reproducibility between labs was also recorded with dilutions of positive ragweed, rye grass, alternaria, milk, house-dust, and mite and birch sera.

Table 2–4 *In Vitro* Test Systems for Detection of Specific IgE Antibody

SYSTEM (MANUFACTURER)	SOLID PHASE	TYPE OF LABEL	RESULTS READ BY
Abbott-Matrix (Abbott Diagnostics)	Membrane	Enzyme	Spectrophotometer
Alatop (Diagnostic Products Corp)	None—liquid phase	Enzyme	Spectrophotometer
Allercoat EAST (Sanofi Diagnostics)	Disc	Enzyme	Spectrophotometer
Allercoat RAST (Sanofi Diagnostics)	Disc	125I	Gamma counter
Allerg*Ens (Dexall Biomedical)	Plastic rod	Enzyme	Spectrophotometer
IgE FAST (Biowhittaker)	Microtiter plate	Enzyme (fluorescence)	Fluorometer
Magic Lite SQ (Ciba Corning)	Micronized paramagnetic particles	Enzyme (chemiluminescence)	Luminometer
MAST-CLA (MAST Immunosystems)	Cellulose thread	Enzyme	Densitometer
Phadebas RAST (Pharmacia Inc.)	Disc	125I	Gamma counter
Phadezyme RAST (Pharmacia Inc.)	Disc	Enzyme (visible product)	Spectrophotometer
Pharmacia ImmunoCAP (Pharmacia Inc.)	Hydrophilic polymer encased in a capsule	Enzyme (fluorescence)	Fluorometer
Ventrex VAST (Hycor Biomedical)	Disc	125I or Enzyme	Gamma counter Gamma counter Spectrophotometer
Ventrex Turbo-VAST (Hycor Biomedical)	Disc	125I	Gamma counter

allergens are adsorbed to the plastic surface by a hydrophobic interaction rather than by the chemical linkages used in the RAST.

An apparent advantage of many of these systems is avoidance of radio-active markers, automation, and a significant reduction in the incubations required; test results are available in from one to three hours. However, these newer technologies frequently give different values from each other.[36–38] These differences may be attributed to a number of factors, such as the potency of the allergens used, the type of solid phase employed, varying adsorption to the plastic surface by the allergens used, and the specificity of the anti-IgE used by the different manufacturers. Of equal importance are the quality control measures taken prior to releasing these assays for clinical and commercial use.

Conclusions

Rapid advances in the development of *in vitro* technology to measure allergen specific IgE antibody continue, and those physicians treating the allergic patient should be prepared to incorporate these changes into practice. However, it is important that we maintain a critical attitude toward forthcoming technology. While the number of commercial kits available to measure specific IgE levels increase, so does the need to evaluate their claims of efficiency in diagnosis.

As with any diagnostic procedure, the use of these procedures should be part of a complete clinical evaluation by a well-informed physician knowledgeable about their limitations. Such physicians should be capable of incorporating this information into responsible, judicious, and effective management of allergic patients.

References

1. Prausnitz C, Kustner J. Studien über die überempfindlichkeit. *Cent Backt* 1921;86:160.
2. Ishizaka K, Ishizaka T, Hornbrook MH. Physicochemical properties of reaginic antibody. V. correlation of reaginic activity with the E-globulin antibody. *J Immunol* 1966;97:840.
3. Johansson SGO. Raised levels of a new immunoglobulin class (IgND) in asthma. *Lancet* 1967;2:951–953.
4. Bennich H, Ishizaka K, Johansson SGO, et al. Immunoglobulin E, a new class of human immunoglobulin. *Bull WHO* 1968;38.
5. Ceska M, Lundkvist U. A new and simple radioimmunoassay method for the determination of IgE. *Immunochemistry* 1972;9:1021.
6. Johansson SGO, Berlund A, Kjellman N. Comparison of IgE values as determined with different solid phase radioimmunoassay methods. *Clin Allergy* 1976;5:91.
7. Wide L, Bennich H, Johansson SGO. Diagnosis of allergy by an *in-vitro* test for allergen antibodies. *Lancet* 1967;2:1105.
8. Evans R, Reisman RE, Wypych JI, et al. An Immunologic evaluation of ragweed sensitive patients by newer techniques. *J Allergy Clin Immunol* 1972;49:285.

9. Aaas K, Lundkvist U. The radioallergosorbent test with a purified allergen from cod fish. *Clin Allerg* 1973;3:255.
10. Eriksson NE. Diagnosis of reaginic allergy with house dust, animal dander and allergens in adult patients. III. Case histories and combinations of case histories, skin tests, and RAST compared with provocation tests. *Int Arch Allergy Appl Immunol* 1977;53:441.
11. Hoffman DR. Dog and cat allergens: urinary proteins or dander proteins. *Ann Allergy* 1980;45:205.
12. Dolovich J, Bell B. Allergy to product(s) of ethylene oxide gas. *J Allergy Clin Immunol* 1978;62:30.
13. Karol MH, Alarie Y. Antigens which detect IgE antibodies in workers sensitive to toluene diisocyanate. *Clin Allergy* 1980;10:101.
14. Norman PS, Lichtenstein LM, Ishizaka K. Diagnostic tests in ragweed hay fever. A comparison of direct skin tests, IgE antibody measurements, and basophil release. *J Allergy Clin Immunol* 1973;52:210–224.
15. Berg TLO, Johansson SGO. Allergy diagnosis with the radioallergosorbent test. A comparison with the results of skin and provocation tests in an unselected group of children with asthma and hayfever. *J Allergy Clin Immunol* 1974;54:209.
16. Welsh PW, Yunginger JW, Kern EB, et al. Preseasonal IgE Ragweed antibody level as a predictor of response to therapy of ragweed hay fever with intranasal cromolyn sodium solution. *J Allergy Clin Immunol* 1977;60:104.
17. Council on Scientific Affairs (AMA). *In vitro* testing for allergy. Report II of the allergy panel. *JAMA* 1987;258:1639.
18. Lundkvist U. Research and development of the RAST technology. In Evans R, ed. *Advances in Diagnosis of Allergy: RAST.* 1975;85–99.
19. Gleich GJ, Yunginger JW. The radioallergosorbent test: Its present place and likely future in the practice of allergy. *Advances Asthma and Allergy* 1975;2:1.
20. Deuschl H, Johansson SGO. Specific IgE antibodies in nasal secretion from patients with allergic rhinitis and with a negative or weakly positive RAST on the serum. *Clinical Allergy* 1977;7:195–202.
21. Nalebuff DJ. Letter to the editor. *Clinical Allergy* 1978;8:99–100.
22. Nalebuff DJ, Fadal RG, Ali M. The study of IgE in the diagnosis of allergic disorders in an otoloarynlogy practice. *Otolaryngol Head Neck Surg* 1978;87:351–358.
23. Nalebuff DJ. An enthusiastic view of the use of RAST in clinical allergy. *Immunology and Allergy Practice* 1981;3:18.
24. Nalebuff DJ. *In vitro* Testing methodologies: Evolution and Current Status. *Otolaryngol Clin N Amer (Otolarngic Allergy)* 1992;25:27–41.
25. Hoffman DR. Comparison of methods of performing the radioallergosorbent test: Phadebas, Fadal–Nalebuff and Hoffman procedures. *Ann Allergy* 1980;45:343.
26. De Filippi I, Yman L, Schroder H. Clinical accuracy of updated version the Phadebas RAST Test. *Ann Allergy* 1981;46:249.
27. American Academy of Allergy and Immunology/Committee on In Vitro tests 1981 study. This unpublished data is available from the author on request.
28. Kelso JM, Sodhi N, Gosselin VA, Yunginger JW. Diagnostic performance characteristics of the standard Phadebas RAST, modified RAST, and Pharmacia CAP system versus skin testing. *Ann Allergy* 1991;67:511–14.
29. Dolen WK, Williams PB, Koepke JW, Seiner JC. Immunoassay of specific IgE: low level assays require measurement of allergen specific assay background. *Ann Allergy* 1992;69:151–156.
30. Miller SP, Marinkovich VA, Riege DH, et al. Application of the MAST immunodiagnostic system to the determination of allergen-specific IgE. *Clin Chem* 1984;30:1467–1472.
31. Seltzer JM, Halpern GM, Tsay YG, et al. Correlation of allergy test results obtained by the FAST, RAST, and prick-puncture methods. *Ann Allergy* 1985;54:25.
32. Metzel PS, Morris N. A new chemiluminescence immunoassay system. *Am Clin Prod Rev,* May 1986.
33. Connell JT. A comparison of Acti*tip Allerg*E and Allerg*ENS system ti Phadebas RAST and Phadebas IgE Prist in assaying total IgE and Specific IgE in human serum. *Amer J Rhinology* 1988;2:135.
34. Axen R, Drevin H, Kober A, Yman L. A new laboratory diagnostic system applied to allergy

testing. In Johansson SGO, ed. Clinical Workshop. IgE Antibodies and the Pharmacia CAP System in Allergy Diagnosis. Uppsala 1988:3–7.

35. Law SJ, Miller T, Piran U, et al. Novel poly-substituted aryl acridium esters and their use in immunoassay. *J Bioluminescence* 1989;4:88–89.

36. Perelmutter L, Emanuel I. Assessment of *in vitro* IgE testing to diagnose allergic disease. *Ann Allergy* 1985;55:762.

37. Emanuel I. Comparison of *in vitro* allergy diagnostic methods. *Immunol Allergy Practice* 1985;7:10–483.

38. Pecoud A, Peitrequin R, Fasel J, et al. Comparison of two assays for the determination of specific IgE in serum of atopic and nonatopic subjects: the Allergenetics FAST and the Phadezym RAST. *Allergy* 1986;41(4):243–249.

· 3 ·

Performance Characteristics in the Evaluation of In Vitro Assays

IVOR EMANUEL, M.D.
LEWIS L. PERELMUTTER, PH.D.

The ideal qualities for any laboratory procedure are:

- sensitivity
- specificity
- overall efficiency
- excellent predictive value
- reproducible
- quantitative
- safe
- inexpensive
- ease of use
- fast

These qualities should be the goals for both the manufacturers and users of assays to detect specific immunoglobulin E (IgE) antibodies against various allergens. Of the above, sensitivity, specificity, overall efficiency, predictive value, and reproducibility are considered the most important performance characteristics of *in vitro* allergy procedures. Furthermore, several of the above parameters are used for quality assurance and quality control (QA/QC)

31

for daily use of the procedures, FDA approval of a test kit, intralaboratory comparison of test methodologies and interlaboratory evaluation, that is, the College of American Pathologists.

In the clinical use of any diagnostic test, the key element is its predictive value (PV), the ability of the test to discriminate between health and the disease state it is intended to establish. The predictive value of any test is dependent on the quality of its sensitivity and specificity, as well as the prevalence of the disease under study in the population being investigated. Disease prevalence should not be confused with the rate of occurrence or disease incidence. A chronic disease with a low incidence, for example, may still be widespread or prevalent due to the long period of time the disease exists in those adversely affected. For a laboratory test, sensitivity can be defined as a positive test in diseased patients; specificity is negative tests in healthy patients. In this chapter, we will consider the role that these factors play in the statistical aspect of diagnostic test results within the broad context of their usefulness in the practice of medicine. We will also try to illustrate these principles by constructing models of the *in vivo* diagnostic skin test and the *in vitro* assay for specific IgE in the clinical practice of allergy.

Sensitivity and Specificity

When evaluating the quality of a given diagnostic test, its sensitivity can be calculated as follows. When the patient is known to suffer from a given disease and a diagnostic test for that disease is positive, the result is referred to as true-positive (TP). False-negatives (FN) are negative test results obtained from patients known to have the disease in question. A simple formula for determining the sensitivity of the test is to divide the number of true-positives by the number of diseased patients (true-positives plus false-negatives) and multiply by 100 (Table 3–1).

The determination of the specificity of a given diagnostic test is equally straightforward. When the test results obtained in healthy individuals are positive, they are designated as false-positive (FP). The negative test results produced in a healthy individual are regarded as true-negatives (TN). To calculate the specificity of the test, again, it is only necessary to divide the number of true-negatives by the total number of healthy individuals (true-negatives plus false-positives) and multiply by 100 (Table 3–1).

Overall efficiency of a laboratory test result combines the definitions of sensitivity and specificity (Table 3–2).

Since overall efficiency is a blend of the specificity and sensitivity of an assay, it reflects best its performance relative to health and disease in a population.

The predictive value of a positive result can be determined by dividing the number of true-positives by the total number of positive results (Table 3–1) or

Table 3-1 Laboratory Test Result*

PREVALENCE (%)	POSITIVE	NEGATIVE	CHARACTERISTIC (%)
Number sick	True-positive (TP)	False-negative (FN)	Sensitivity $= \dfrac{\text{TP}}{\text{TP} + \text{FN}} \times 100$
Number well	False-positive (FP)	True-negative (TN)	Specificity $= \dfrac{\text{TN}}{\text{TN} + \text{FP}} \times 100$
Total Patients			Predictive value $=$ Positive result $\dfrac{\text{TP}}{\text{TP} + \text{FP}} \times 100$

*By arranging data as shown, one can determine test qualities of sensitivity (positive) in disease, specificity (negativity in health), and the predictive value of a positive result (the likelihood of the disease).

**Table 3–2   Overall Efficiency
of a Laboratory Procedure**

Overall efficiency = sensitivity + specificity

$$\text{Efficiency} = \frac{\text{Tp} + \text{TN}}{\text{TP} + \text{FP} + \text{TN} + \text{FN}} \times 100$$

by using Bayes' formula, first described in 1763 in the essay: "Toward Solving a Problem in the Doctrine of Chance"[1] (Table 3–3).

When performing a single laboratory test, the disease prevalence may be more important than either its sensitivity or its specificity in determining the predictive value of a positive result (i.e., the likelihood of disease). Using Bayes' formula, for example, note the change in predictive value obtained as the prevalence of disease is increased from 1% to 10%. Improving the laboratory test's specificity by increasing its confidence limit to 99% also significantly improves the ultimate predictive value, especially when the disease prevalence is relatively low.

Cutoff Point

With quantitative tests, it is possible to vary both sensitivity and specificity by changing the cutoff level at which the test is considered positive. It is customary, although arbitrary, to use 2 SD above the mean value of normal controls as the cutoff point to obtain a 95% specificity. (A level of 1.5 × negative control binding is used in the modified RAST (mRAST).) The specificity can be increased to 99% by widening the range of normal to 3 SD above the mean value of normal controls (twice the binding of negative controls in the Modified RAST). Thus, the customary cutoff point can be altered to produce a very specific test, with rare false-positive results, or to produce an extremely sensitive test, with rare false-negative results.[2]

Table 3–3   Bayes' Theorem

$$PV = \frac{P \times Se}{(P \times Se) + (1 - P)(1 - Sp)}$$

PV, the predictive value of the positive result (i.e., the likelihood of disease); P, disease prevalence; Se, sensitivity (proportion of diseased persons who give positive results); and Sp, the specificity (proportion of healthy persons who give negative results).

False-Positives in an Allergy Workup

While the implications of missing a clinically relevant disease due to a false-negative result are clear, less obvious is the mischief that derives from the occurrence of a small percentage of false-positive results; this problem becomes particularly acute when performing multiple independent tests, as is often done in an allergic work-up.[2] If the patient is indeed normal, the more times he is tested, the greater the chance he will be classified abnormal in at least one of the tests performed. If there is only one test done, the 95% confidence limit is adequate.[3] If, however, one performs two independent tests on the same normal patient, then a 97% confidence limit must be used to ensure adequate specificity; the probability that both tests will be in the normal range is 0.97×0.97, which gives a product of 0.95. When 15 independent tests are done in a normal individual using a test with a 95% confidence limit, there is less than an even chance that all the results will be in the normal range (Table 3–3). Changing the cutoff point to create a 99% confidence limit (widening the range of normal to 3 SD above the means of negative controls) solves this problem; if one does 15 such independent tests on a group of normal individuals, only 3% of the patients will be declared abnormal in one of the tests in the battery (2).

The following are examples of statistical principles used for RAST and skin test analysis.

Example 1

Twenty-eight patients with definite allergic reactions after cat or dog exposure were studied and reported by Wüthrich and Arrendal (1979).[4] Eight of these patients had a clinical history of specific allergy to dog and not to cat; the remaining 20 had clear-cut history of allergy to cat and not to dog. Each patient was tested for skin reactivity (prick test) and when negative, followed up by an intracutaneous skin test at an allergen concentration of 1:1000 weight/volume (w/v) to both allergens. In addition, all patients' sera were examined for the presence or absence of specific IgE antibodies against either allergen; a total of 112 laboratory tests were performed. By arranging the data in an appropriate form, it can be shown that the complete skin test, while 100% sensitive, was only 70% specific; the Phadebas RAST, on the other hand, was 100% specific but only 70% sensitive. The predictive value of the positive test result was 100% for the Phadebas RAST and 80% for the skin test. In this report sickness and health were determined primarily by history and confirmed by provocation test (Table 3–4).

Example 2

In a paper by Bryant et al.,[5] 612 bronchial provocations were done in 153 asthmatic patients; each patient was tested against four allergens (*Dermato*

Table 3–4   Sensitivity, Specificity, and Predictive Values

Prevalence (50%)	PHADEBAS RAST	+	−	Characteristic (%)	
History	+28	22	6	Sensitivity	80
plus					
Provocation	−28	0	28	Specificity	100
Total	56	22	34	Predictive Value + Result	100

Prevalence (50%)	COMPLETE SKIN TEST	+	−	Characteristic (%)	
History	+28	28	0	Sensitivity	100
plus					
Provocation	−28	8	20	Specificity	70
Total	56	36	20	Predictive Value + Result	80

phagoides pteronyssinus, rye grass, plantain, and *A. fumagatus*). Using provocation results as the benchmark for the presence or absence of specific disease, these investigators compared the results of the skin and the RAST tests. All 110 patients with positive bronchial provocation tests to *D. pteronyssinus* had some skin reactivity to the homologous allergen; there were 91 positives and 19 equivocal skin test results. When tested with the RAST procedure, 91% gave positive results (more than twice the binding of negative controls). By contrast, among 43 patients with negative provocation tests to *D. pteronyssinus*, 11 had some skin reactivity but only one was positive by the RAST procedure. Thus the RAST had excellent sensitivity and specificity and far surpassed the skin test in predictive value. The predictive value of the skin test depended on whether the equivocal results were included as positive or negative. By including them with the clear-cut positives, the test assumed 100% sensitivity; however, specificity fell to 75%. On the other hand, when the equivocals were included among the negative test results, the test qualities reversed and sensitivity fell to 80% while the specificity matched RAST (Table 3–4).

More recent studies have evaluated *in vitro* technologies.[6,7] Kelso et al.[8] reported results from three *in vitro* assays for allergen-specific IgE, the standard Phadebas radioallergosorbent test (PhRAST), mRAST, and the new Pharmacia CAP System (CAP) were compared with skin prick testing (SPT) results in 104 patients with allergic rhinitis and/or asthma, and 24 nonatopic controls. Five allergens were evaluated: cat, *D. pteronyssinus*, Alternaria, June grass, and short ragweed. Using SPT results as the reference standard, the PhRAST had the lowest sensitivity (62%) and highest specificity (99%). The CAP achieved higher sensitivity (87%). The overall frequency of positive results in controls was 0% for PhRAST, 1.7% for CAP, and 3.3% for mRAST. If the threshold for a positive mRast was raised to ≥ class 2, this assay achieved performance characteristics similar to the CAP. According to Kelso et al.,[8] if the results of these *in vitro* tests are used as the sole guide to the prescription of environmental control and immunotherapy in unselected patients with rhinitis and asthma, the performance characteristics of the CAP make it the preferred test.

In addition, Bousquet et al.[9] did a comparison between PhRAST and Pharmacia CAP system in 106 unselected patients. These patients had a detailed clinical history and skin prick tests with standardized allergen extracts. IgE to cat, *D. pteronyssinus*, Alternaria, orchard grass, olive, and Parietaria pollen were tested; 470 tests were run. The specificity, sensitivity, and overall efficiency of both *in vitro* tests ranged from 85.5% to 100% except for olive pollen, in which the sensitivity of both *in vitro* tests was low (68.2% for the new test and 63.6% for RAST). Except for orchard grass pollen, the sensitivity and specificity of CAP were better than that of RAST. There was a highly significant correlation between both tests (r range 0.864 to 0.987). Bousquet et al.[9] concluded that CAP competes favorably with PhRAST and has the advantage of being automated and eliciting results in kilounits per liter.

Thus, the ability to perform comparison studies between *in vitro* allergy systems or against provocation and/or skin tests allows the evaluation of a given system. This usually results in improvements in the assay and an understanding of the factors that influence assays to detect specific IgE response.[10] Such factors are described below.

Allergens Attached to Solid Supports Used in In Vitro Methods for the Measurement of Specific IgE

The term "allergen," as commonly used, refers to a mixture of chemical components extracted from an allergenic complex such as pollen. Ragweed allergen, a complex of chemical components, has been shown to be a mixture of ragweed antigens including E, K, RA3-RA6, and phospholipase. Each of the purified components of the mixture is also referred to as an allergen. All allergens give rise to antibodies of the IgE class, and most allergens also induce other classes of immunoglobulins. The amount of IgE and nature of the response to the allergen is controlled by the genotype of that individual, the amount of allergen the person is exposed to, and the route of exposure. Allergens range in size from 5–70 kD with the majority (75%) being between 10 to 40 kD. These compounds are easily absorbed through mucous membranes and give rise to IgE biosynthesis. Most allergens, because of their complexity and relatively high molecular weight, have many and varied immunodeterminants (allergic determinants or epitopes) on their surface. Epitopes are the portion of the antigen to which the antibody is directed. They serve as the cross-linking sites for the binding of bivalent IgE molecules on the surface of cells. Many of these allergenic substances are acidic proteins with isoelectric points of 4 to 6. These allergenic proteins are mainly globular in nature, and they frequently are readily extractable and in greater abundance than the other proteins in the extract. They are extremely efficient in the induction of IgE antibodies. Within any allergenic extract, there are often many components. Some of these components are considered to be *major* allergens, defined as a purified component to which 60% of the skin test positive patients have shown specific IgE antibodies. Extracts also contain minor allergens, defined as purified allergenic components of a crude extract that bind IgE in less than 10% of the skin-test-positive patients. The minor allergens include both acidic and basic proteins and have a broader molecular weight range.

Many pollens from related plants, as well as other related allergen sources, usually contain some identical proteins, as well as different proteins sharing similar allergenic determinants. They may also contain unique proteins with unique allergenic determinants, which could differentiate them from other species in the same family. Knowledge of the degree and type of shared and/or unique allergenic determinants acquired from allergenic cross-reactivity studies may lead to the production of more effective allergens for use in *in vitro* technology.

Unfortunately, manufacturers of kits for specific IgE do not necessarily use the same allergen source for a particular allergen, nor do they extract or purify the material in exactly the same way. The solid supports used to bind the allergen also differ from company to company. The solid supports differ in the type of allergen preferentially bound as well as the amount of each allergen bound from an extract. Those solid supports are polysaccharides activated by cyanogen bromide, depend upon free amino groups in the allergens for linkage. Some allergenic substances found in extracts do not lend themselves to this type of reaction. Certain allergens are not readily adsorbed onto the surface of polystyrene but might attach strongly to polyvinylchloride. One can surmise from the above that major differences can and do exist between commercial assay kits even for the same allergen.

The allergens placed on the solid support for use in *in vitro* specific IgE measurements should contain all of the pertinent allergenic components of a mixture. Allergic individuals who are reactive only to some of the minor allergenic components could easily be missed if the extract on the solid support lacked these components. Efforts to insure that all relevant allergenic substances in an extract are reflected on the solid supports have been tested using pooled serum from allergic patients sensitive to a particular allergen. Demonstration that the allergen fixed to the solid would adsorb out the specific IgE to that allergen is taken as evidence that the pertinent allergenic substances are indeed linked to the solid support.

The problems of different allergen sources, different extraction schemes, different purification procedures, and different solid supports used to bind the allergens for *in vitro* assays for specific IgE, make it unlikely that results with one kit would be comparable to another type of kit even for the same allergen. Unlikely as it may seem, from our prior observations, some kits for specific allergens from manufacturers do show comparable results as demonstrated by CAP evaluation.

The problems alluded to for allergens used in *in vitro* assays also hold for skin test allergens as well. Allergens, if they are to be compared from one lab or clinic to the next, using *in vitro* technologies, patient skin testing, or any other *in vivo* techniques must be characterized, purified and standardized. This need becomes even more acute if one attempts to correlate *in vivo* measurements with results obtained with *in vitro* procedures. Quality control by the allergen supplies of each extract for both *in vivo* and *in vitro* techniques must also be standardized using appropriate biological activity assays and/or relevant electrophoretic immunoblotting and immunoelectrophoretic techniques capable of characterizing and quantifying each allergen in a given extract.

The manufacturers of systems for the measurement of specific IgE must likewise have a quality control program in place that insures all appropriate allergens are linked to their particular solid support.

Specific IgE Contained in the Patient's Serum

In considering the measurement of specific IgE binding to a particular allergen in an *in vitro* assay, one must take into consideration the nature of the IgE contained in the patient's serum. When one measures patient IgE to a specific allergen, we are essentially dealing with two variables. One variable is the affinity (avidity) of the patient's IgE for the particular immunodeterminants contained on the solid support. A patient with a high affinity (avidity) antibody will show binding even when IgE concentrations are moderately low, while a patient with a lower affinity (avidity) but with the same concentration of antibodies will have less IgE bound to the fixed antigen on the solid support. In reality, then, we are measuring two distinct conditions when we measure specific IgE. We are measuring the concentration of IgE contained in the patient's sera as well as the affinity (avidity) of that IgE for a particular allergen. Therefore, a quantitative measurement of the patient's IgE is sometimes difficult to achieve, and comparison of results from one kit to another becomes difficult due to these differences.

Specific IgE measurements are also prone to interference by other classes of immunoglobulins. Allergens, as previously noted, induce not only IgE but also immunoglobulin G (IgG) and other immunoglobulins.[11] IgG antibody especially could interfere with determinations of specific IgE by steric hindrance or by competing for the same binding site, if it is specific for the same immunodeterminant on the allergen as the IgE. These interferences have been noted,[11] and simple adsorption of the IgG by staph protein A, or better yet, with latex coated beads containing anti-human IgG, can usually remove the interfering antibody.

Nonspecific binding of patient IgE does occur, the extent of which is dependent on the concentration of IgE in the patient's serum (the higher the concentration the more nonspecific binding). The type of solid support also influences nonspecific binding. Some supports are more prone than others to this phenomenon. Finally, the allergen itself can contribute to nonspecific binding. These problems of nonspecific binding can be taken into account and negated through the use of specific reference sera for each allergen as well as appropriate controls.

The Labeled Anti-IgE Molecule Used to Detect Patient Specific IgE

Of critical importance in the determination of patient specific IgE is the labeled anti-human IgE used to detect it. The manufacturers of today's commercial kits all have available to them their own particular anti-human IgE molecules. Some manufacturers use monoclonal anti-human IgE, while the majority use polyclonal anti-human IgE because the average affinity of the polyclonal antibody is usually greater. Affinity of the labeled anti-human IgE determines the amount of IgE that can be detected; the greater the affinity constant, the smaller the amount of IgE that can be accurately measured. More importantly, these anti-human IgE molecules utilize different enzymes, each employing a different substrate. These differences can and do lead to variations between kits. It is essential for the user of these assays to know something of the performance characteristics of each of the commercial kits available. Comparison by various authors of the most popular *in vitro* assays for specific serum IgE antibody[6,7] showed major differences in sensitivities and reproducibilities of each of the assay systems.[6,7] Some of the assay systems definitely were more sensitive than others; but it was pointed out by Perelmutter et al.,[12] after examination of coefficients of variations, that none of the EIA systems examined had sufficient reproducibility to evaluate low end responders, that is, individuals who showed only low levels of binding to the specific allergen.

Quality Control Programs

For any laboratory test, including tests for IgE, a strong quality control program should be put into practice. Recently several manufacturers have supplied standards of serum that reacted against the specific allergens used in the testing rather than the use of one serum to one particular allergen for all comparisons. One may also use serum from patients shown to be allergic to a particular allergen in the past so that a reference stock can be made up for those specific allergens. Negative control sera to determine nonspecific bindings is also essential for accurate testing. It is extremely important that any laboratory doing *in vitro* testing procedures follow a quality control program using appropriate reference standards so that daily standard deviations can be calculated and followed over time.

When quality control programs have been instituted and the various immunoassays have been run according to protocol, the results from *in vitro* specific IgE tests have correlated well with skin prick tests and intradermal testing methods such as Serial End-Point Titration (S.E.T.). Good correlation with other *in vivo* clinical tests such as inhalation testing and other forms of provocative testing has also been shown. The tests have also been correlated with *in vitro* histamine release. Clinically the *in vitro* IgE assay offers many advantages over other *in vitro* techniques, which are, at this point, not nearly as well characterized. Because there are many *in vitro* procedures to measure IgE antibody response and because there are many clinical reference laboratories and procedures used in physicians' offices, there is a need to have a quality control program that sets standards for the *in vitro* allergy user. Thus, the College of American Pathologists (CAP), supported by the leading allergy centers in the United States, developed target values for common allergens for serum specimens. These sera can be employed by all users of *in vitro* allergy tests.

Conclusion

The application of performance characteristics to *in vitro* allergy tests for specific IgE determination has played an important role in the quality of such tests and has improved the capabilities of the user of such tests. The CAP evaluation of various procedures allows each user to evaluate his/her own results with respect to the whole. This evaluation leads to improvements in these assays and elimination of poorly performing tests.

As the technology advances, there will be improvements in better standards; for example, the use of absolute IgE antibody standards. The procedures will go from being qualitative to quantitative. There will be improvements in accuracy, analytical sensitivity, binding capacity of allergens to solid phases, kinetics of antibody–antigen interaction, use of standardized allergens, normalization and elimination of classes to absolute levels of IgE antibody response. With improved reporting systems (CAP, etc.) for proficiency testing, there will be excellent predictive (positive or negative) values for determining IgE-allergic disease.

References

1. Bayes T. An essay toward solving a problem in the doctrine of chance. *Philo Trans Roy Soc* 1763;53:370.
2. Nalebuff DJ, Fadal RG, Ali M. *Predictive Value of Laboratory Tests*. In Fadal RG, Nalebuff DJ, eds. RAST in Clinical Allergy, Symposia Foundation; 1989.
3. Schoen I, Brooks SH. Judgment based on ninety-five percent confidence limits: A statistical dilemma involving multi-test screening and proficiency testing of multiple specimens. *Am J Clin Pathol* 1970;53:190.

4. Wüthrich B, Arrendal H. RAST in the diagnosis of hypersensitivity to dog and cat allergens. *Clin Allergy* 1979;9:191.
5. Bryant DH, Burns NW, Lazarus L. The correlation between skin tests, bronchial provocation tests and serum levels of IgE specific for common allergens in patients with asthma. *Clin Allergy* 1975;5:145.
6. Emanuel I. Comparison of *in-vitro* allergy diagnostic methods. *Immunol Allergy Practice* 1985;7:483.
7. Emanuel I. Comparison of *in-vitro* allergy diagnostic assays. *Ear Nose Throat J*, Jan 1990; vol 69, No. 1.
8. Kelso JM, Sodhi N, Gosselin VA, Yunginger JW. Diagnostic performance characteristics of the standard Phadebas RAST, modified RAST, and Pharmacia CAP system versus skin testing. *Ann Allergy* 1991;67:511.
9. Bousquet J, Chanez P, Chanal I, Michel FB. Comparison between RAST and Pharmacia CAP system: A new automated specific IgE assay. *J Allergy Clin Immunol* 1990;85:1039.
10. Perelmutter L, Emanuel I. Assessment of *in vitro* IgE testing to diagnose allergic disease. *Am Allergy* 1985;55:762.
11. Zimmerman EM, Yunginger TW, Gleich GJ. Interference in ragweed pollen and honeybee venom RAST. *J Allergy Clin Immunol* 1980;66:386.
12. Perelmutter L, Massari M, Mansmann MC Jr. An evaluation of the enzyme immunoassay. *Immunol Allergy Practice* 1991;3:93.

· 4 ·

In Vivo Versus In Vitro Methods of Allergy Evaluation: A Review of the Literature

JACK B. ANON, M.D., F.A.C.S., F.A.A.O.A.

Precise clinical determination of antigen-specific sensitivity has undergone considerable change in recent years. Prior to 1967, *in vivo* techniques were standard procedure for evaluation of patient allergy status and included such provocation tests as direct application of antigen into the conjunctiva, upper airway exposure via nasal challenge or inhalation, and epidermal exposure, by patch test, prick test, or intradermal injection. Subsequent to discovery of the reaginic properties of immunoglobulin E (IgE) in 1967, however, radio-isotope technology was applied to measure antibody response to antigen challenge. Since that time, the radioallergosorbent test (RAST) and newer derivative enzyme-linked immunosorbent assay (ELISA) assays have become widely accepted as viable and effective *in vitro* alternatives to *in vivo* evaluation methods. While such *in vitro* testing has the obvious advantage of avoiding any possible adverse patient reactions, there has been some question about its sensitivity in comparison with *in vivo* methods.

In this chapter, *in vitro* and *in vivo* testing methods are compared by literature review. For the purposes of this discussion, particular attention is given to skin prick and single intradermal tests, as the *in vivo* methods most commonly used by general allergists; the correlation between *in vitro* testing and serial endpoint titration is addressed in Chapter 5. Similarly, RAST is presented as the prototypic *in vitro* test. It should be kept in mind, however, that many new technologies are currently available and others are forthcoming. Enzyme techniques, for example, are discussed in five chapters in this book. Many of the conclusions drawn about *in vitro* technology in general may be extrapolated to include these newer methods. Finally, it should be noted that the scratch test is no longer recommended by the AMA Council on Scientific Affairs and is consequently not discussed here.

Introduction to *In Vivo* Testing

In vivo testing measures a patient's degree of sensitivity to an antigen by evaluating the IgE reactivity of a small test area, which can be assumed to predict the patient's overall IgE response.

Pretest Considerations

Before initiating any skin test, both positive and negative control tests must be conducted to establish the patient's capability for appropriate response to antigen challenge. For negative control, the diluent normally used for skin testing is used without the active antigen. A positive response to this challenge implies the presence of dermatographism, which would significantly complicate the evaluation of results from further skin testing. The positive control test utilizes the universal-allergen properties of histamine. If there is no wheal response to a 1 mg/mL histamine challenge, the patient may have taken an antihistamine, which would block the skin's normal reactivity, and testing should be postponed. Poorly reactive skin, as in the elderly patient, can lead to the same findings.

Testing Procedures: Prick and Intradermal Skin Tests

The prick test is an epicutaneous evaluation method involving the introduction of a small sample (usually about 3×10^{-6} mL) of concentrated antigen (commonly, 1:10 w/v or 1:20 w/v) into the most superficial layer of skin. The small amount of active antigen used minimizes the risk of a constitutional reaction.

One technique for prick testing is the Pepys method, in which a drop of test antigen is placed on the back or volar surface of the arm. A #26 needle is then passed through the drop and the epicutaneous layer of skin is lifted, allowing the antigen to enter the broken skin. After approximately 15 minutes, the resulting wheal size is measured and graded according to various scales. The primary drawback to this method is its lack of reproducibility, given the potentially variable amount of antigen introduced into the skin from one test to another, even in the same patient, and among different investigators.

In a consequential search for improved standardization of prick test methods, the Morrow-Brown needle was developed. This metal or plastic disposable needle was originally designed at a length of 1 mm but was recently lengthened to 1.6 mm and made triangular in shape. With this device, the tester places a drop of antigen as before and plunges the Morrow-Brown needle, held at a 90° angle, through the drop and into the epidermis. After 15 minutes, the resulting wheal is measured against a scale based on the patient's baseline histamine response, defined as 3+. Thus, an antigen-response wheal of similar size also is considered to be 3+, a wheal larger than the control response is measured at 4+, and wheals one-third or two-thirds the size of the histamine response are 1+ and 2+, respectively.

Other prick devices have been developed, but a detailed account of each is beyond the scope of this chapter.

Single intradermal testing is the other *in vivo* method most commonly used for allergy evaluation. Following an initial prick test yielding negative or equivocal results, indicating that the patient does not have a high degree of sensitivity to the trial antigen, a single intradermal skin test is employed. This technique involves injection of a small quantity (.01 to .02 mL) of dilute antigen (commonly, 1:1000 or 1:500 w/v) into the deeper layer of skin and allows for more precise and reproducible introduction of the test antigen. Various scales are used to measure the resulting wheal and flare response, depending on the preference of the investigator.

Intradermal testing is an extremely sensitive technique, although the clinical relevance of its increased sensitivity has been questioned, given that such a high level of skin test sensitivity may in fact lead to "biologically false-positive results" that may not bear a relationship to clinical disease.

In Vitro Testing

RAST is the most familiar *in vitro* method currently available and is used here as a standard for comparison. It should be noted, however, that the conventional Phadebas radioallergosorbent test (phRAST) has been modified in several key ways, described in detail in two chapters in this book. One major change of the Fadal-Nalebuff modified RAST (mRAST), made in response to an unacceptably high rate of false-negative results, was lowering the cutoff point for definition of sensitivity. This change has yielded a test that is more sensitive than the phRAST while remaining highly specific. Nevertheless, most comparisons in the literature reflect data from the phRAST, and the differences between the two should be kept in mind when comparing *in vitro* and *in vivo* test results.

Comparability of *In Vivo* and *In Vitro* Allergy Testing

While *in vivo* techniques are generally agreed to be the more sensitive means of allergy assessment, the advantages of *in vitro* methods have been widely discussed and include greater stability of the *in vitro* test antigen, which is securely attached to a solid matrix; no risk of systemic reaction; and nonreactivity both to concomitantly used medications and to the presence of dermatographism. In addition, the position statement of the American Academy of Allergy and Immunology[1] favorably compares the sensitivity and specificity of *in vitro* vs *in vivo* tests.

Generally, when skin testing is compared with various *in vitro* testing methods, data are reasonably well correlated. The most commonly reported discrepancy involves a positive skin test coupled with a negative *in vitro* test, although most studies also report positive *in vitro* results with negative skin tests.

An editorial by Kniker[2] explored the *in vitro* vs *in vivo* relationship and clarifies some of the common problems encountered in comparing the two. He pointed out, for example, that study populations should have similar degrees of sensitivity and that positive skin reactions should be reasonably well defined. In addition, he noted that testing requires either well characterized and standard extracts, or that the same lot of antigen used for skin testing also be used for the *in vitro* test. Kniker concluded that modern literature should focus on issues of quality assurance rather than the continual search for the merits of one test modality vs the other.

In Vivo vs *In Vitro* Allergy Testing: Clinical Experience

Many comparisons of *in vitro* and *in vivo* study results have been made in the literature. As early as 1973, for example, Stenius[3] studied 31 patients with rhinitis, evaluated by prick and intradermal testing with *Dermatophagoides pteronyssinus*. Both tests used serial dilutions of antigen, beginning with a weaker concentration and progressing to more concentrated solutions. Nasal provocation also was performed, as was phRAST testing for specific IgE antibody. Seventeen patients had a positive phRAST score, and concordance between phRAST and skin tests were seen with concentrations of 10^{-5} g/mL. Discordance, when it occurred, was seen at weaker concentrations, as a positive phRAST score accompanied by a negative skin test and, at stronger concentrations (10^{-4} g/mL and higher), as positive skin tests associated with negative phRAST scores. Stenius stated that "... the RAST method of estimating IgE in serum may not be sensitive enough. ..." As noted, however, this is known to have been a major fault of the phRAST system, and the test has since been modified to overcome the problem. Of interest, this author also reported that the nasal provocation test did not correlate with either the skin tests or the *in vitro* test. Recognizing that this was in contradiction to the literature, he proposed several possibilities that could have led to inaccurate results, including errors in antigen delivery to the nose.

Norman et al[4] studied 87 subjects, most of whom had been previously found to have high correlation between skin tests (intradermal injections on the back using tenfold dilutions) and basophil–histamine release to ragweed antigen. For this study, patient sera was stored and specific immunoglobulin E (IgE) antibody response to the same ragweed protein was evaluated. Some of the patients had poor histamine release but demonstrated a positive skin test to the antigen challenge. Interestingly, these same patients tended to manifest fewer symptoms during the ragweed season. In the same fashion, several patients were identified who exhibited no IgE response to ragweed challenge, yet had a positive skin test to weak concentrations of extract. Following analysis of all data, the authors concluded that *in vitro* and *in vivo* tests are clinically equivalent, and that features such as cost and convenience should be considered in determining the appropriate type of test for the individual patient. These investigators also noted that borderline cases require additional clinical data before the proper course of action can be decided.

In a study conducted by Berg and Johansson,[5] 118 children underwent prick, provocation, and RAST analysis for dog, cat, horse, cow, birch, and timothy grass sensitivity. Intradermal testing also was carried out in a select group and, for control purposes, 100 blood samples were studied from a separate group of subjects with no allergic history. Results of phRAST and provocation testing were similar in 76% of cases, while comparison of agreement among phRAST, prick, and provocation results varied with the test antigen. Correlation between positive phRAST and prick scores ranged from 66% to 88% and increased with the degree of response to the prick test. A negative prick test was mirrored by a negative phRAST score in 90% of cases, while 37% of positive prick tests could not be correlated with a positive reaction to provocative challenge. No false-positives were identified with phRAST, but positive intradermal response was associated with negative phRAST and prick test results in 16% of cases. The authors concluded that based on this study, phRAST testing is a useful tool, but they went on to recommend that additional prick testing may be useful in selected cases.

Ahlstedt[6] compared results of intradermal, provocation, and phRAST testing for birch, timothy grass, and/or dog epithelium sensitivity in 65 patients with asthma or allergic rhinitis. The same batches of antigen were used for all tests, and intradermal testing was conducted by titration methods. PhRAST results were scored on a 0 to 4 class scale based on fivefold dilutions of reference serum and recording counts every 2 minutes. Comparison of skin test and phRAST results showed a correlation between positive phRAST (class 2 to 4) and positive intradermal tests in 100% of cases. At the equivocal level (phRAST 1), 43% of cases appeared as a negative intradermal score, and 18% were positive on intradermal testing. These results illustrate the inherent problem with this type of phRAST scoring, rather than with the test itself. Provocation study results reflected those attained with phRAST in 46% of negative cases; 1% of negative phRAST scores were positive on provocation. Equivocal phRAST scores were negative in 46% and positive in 15% of provocation studies. Finally, positive phRAST correlated well with provocation response, with 84% of cases showing agreement between results by the two methods. In a further comparison that included case history as well as skin and provocation test results vs phRAST, these authors found up to a 94% correlation between phRAST results and clinical history indicative of "probable allergy."

Perera et al.[7] looked at several groups of patients to determine the predictive value of phRAST. Group 1 comprised 30 subjects with a three-season history of ragweed hay fever and all with a positive scratch test to short ragweed. Group 2 included 40 patients who underwent rapid preseason immunotherapy following two years of previously untreated symptoms of ragweed allergy. There were 54 patients in Group 3, all of whom had been referred to the practice with a general diagnosis of allergy, and many with asthma as well. The final group of 324 patients had been classified according to history as definitely, equivocally, or not allergic. All patients underwent phRAST evaluation, interpreted on a 0 to 4 scale, where a score of 4 was defined as counts greater than or equal to counts determined for a 1:1 dilution of reference serum. The authors found a 93% correlation between nasal provocation and phRAST in Group 1. In Group 2, where patients had undergone rush immunotherapy, there was a significant inverse correlation between the amount of antigen tolerated and the phRAST score. Obviously, the higher the degree of sensitivity, the less antigen challenge the patient will tolerate. Group 3 patients had skin testing performed by titration intradermally, and none of those with a negative skin test had a positive phRAST. Evaluation of Group 4 revealed a 60% concordance between phRAST and intradermal testing. The investigators subsequently concluded that provocation testing is not indicated in a phRAST-positive patient and that lack of correlation between intradermal and phRAST scores may be more attributable to a false-positive skin test than to a lack of phRAST sensitivity. They further suggested that patients with high phRAST scores begin immunotherapy at low doses and progress carefully. Finally, it was noted that the specificity of phRAST vs skin testing improves the physician's ability to determine the presence of allergic disease.

Considering other types of skin testing, however, Bryant et al[8] looked at 153 asthmatic patients. Prick tests for sensitivity to *D. pteronyssinus*, rye grass, plantain, and *Aspergillus fumigatus* were performed at four different concentrations. Bronchial provocation also was carried out, along with phRAST. The authors concluded that the measurement of specific IgE should not replace the skin prick test. More than a decade later, Bryant's data were carefully reexamined by Nalebuff, Fadal, and Ali,[9] who demonstrated that when

Bryant's prevalence rate is adjusted and sensitivity and specificity are maintained at a constant, the positive predictive value of the skin test drops considerably to 44%, whereby the positive predictive value for phRAST rises dramatically to 96%. Their reinterpretation is attributable to the finding that Bryant's study defined equivocal skin test results as positive when sensitivity was measured but did not include equivocal results in calculations of specificity. In their retrospective analysis, Nalebuff and co-workers aptly pointed out that the clinician must be acutely aware of the concepts of sensitivity (defined as positivity in disease) and specificity (defined as negativity in health) in diagnostic testing. With regards to phRAST, each of these qualities changes in response to the cutoff point for positivity. They further noted that low specificity tests translate into a high rate of false-positive results and may lead to overtreatment of patients.

Recognizing the need for a safer test for patients who had previously exhibited an anaphylactic reaction to penicillin, Kraft and Wide (1976) initiated a study to evaluate testing for antibiotic-allergic patients. Skin tests using penicilloyl-polylsine were compared to benzyl-penicilloyl specific RAST (Wide, Bennich, Johansson technique), and the authors found a 95% correlation. Based on their findings, they recommended that all of the antigenic proteins be included in the RAST.

In a comparative trial undertaken by Reddy et al (1978), 53 patients with several years of rhinitis were compared with 13 controls. All patients underwent allergy screening by prick, intradermal, nasal provocation, leukocyte-histamine release tests, and phRAST (pharmacia scoring 1 to 4+). Patients were divided into three groups. The first group included those with positive history, negative prick test, and variable positive intradermal tests. Patients in the second group had a positive history with positive prick tests to several antigens, and the third group was made up of control subjects. These researchers confirmed a strong correlation between the less sensitive prick test and this type of phRAST (12 of 19 positive prick tests were found to be phRAST-positive as well), and a poor correlation was found between intradermal testing and phRAST. As would be expected, phRAST was 100% specific for the control group.

Of 311 subjects evaluated by questionnaire in 1979, Brown et al (1979) identified 157 who were allergic and 154 who were not. A comparison of prick test, single intradermal test, and phRAST to Bermuda grass revealed a significant correlation between both positive and negative prick tests and phRAST scores. Specifically, 79% of patients with a positive prick test also had a positive phRAST score, and 98% of prick-negative patients had a negative phRAST score. Discrepancies occurred as a small positive prick reaction associated with a negative phRAST. A prick-positive wheal less than 5 mm wide yielded a positive phRAST in 51% of cases, while a prick response of 5 mm or greater yielded a positive phRAST in 91%. In contrast, results of the comparison between single intradermal testing and phRAST was not as close. Only two of 50 individuals with a positive intradermal test also had a positive phRAST. The authors felt that this finding underscored the fact that intradermal testing is nonspecific and yields too many false-positives. Again, however, it should be kept in mind that the cutoff for phRAST is such that low-level positive reactions are inherently missed, and the correlation between the small-wheal prick result would be different if the modified RAST was employed.

Fadal and Nalebuff (1979) studied a population of 80 patients with allergic symptoms and elevated IgE levels. Evaluation studies included skin prick, intradermal, phRAST and, though results will not be addressed here, the scratch test. A positive prick test was found to agree with a positive phRAST in 86% of studies, while negative results of the two agreed in only 39%. For intradermal testing where fivefold dilutions were used, correlation between phRAST and intradermal results depended on the definition of a positive endpoint. When a 1:12,500 dilution was used as the cutoff figure, then there were no false-positive intradermal vs phRAST results, but false-negatives increased from 0 to 60%. These authors, considering the *in vitro* test as their gold standard for valuation of skin test results, concluded that the intradermal test was a reliable alternative.

Vanto et al (1990) studied a group of 164 asthmatic children who underwent prick testing as well as provocation either by bronchial challenge or conjunctival exposure to dog dander. PhRAST also was performed for comparison. Three batches of allergen from different sources were used for the *in vivo* tests, and a positive provocation test was identified in 72 of 164 exposed subjects. Skin prick response correlated with provocation test results in an average of 83% of cases for all three batches of antigen. Agreement between provocation and phRAST also was significant with all antigens but one, which had been identified by the authors as biologically weak and responsible for some inaccurate study results.

Menardo et al (1982) looked at the Morrow-Brown needle, multi-test, modified prick, and single intradermal skin tests vs phRAST tested with *D. pteronyssinus*. High correlation values were documented among all of the methods ($P = 0.996$ to 0.95), but the lowest correlation value was for intradermal testing.

Bousquet et al (1987) conducted a study of 44 patients with grass-season nasal symptoms and positive threefold dilution prick test to orchard grass pollen, with positive IgE levels to the same antigen, as determined by phRAST. Nasal provocation testing performed with active antigen and placebo identified 3 of the 44 whose lack of response was felt to be secondary to differences in mast cell distribution between the skin and the nose. This discrepancy between IgE levels and *in vivo* evidence also had been addressed in 1975 by Huggins and Brostoff, who demonstrated that despite a high correlation among phRAST, prick test, and nasal provocation, the degree of *in vivo* sensitivity did not correspond with the level of IgE found in the sera. These authors postulated that the level of antigen that triggers the release of mediators from mast cells and basophils may differ from the actual serum level of IgE.

Van der Zee et al (1988) identified discrepancies in agreement between phRAST and intracutaneous tests; as is common, disagreement usually took the form of a positive skin test that was not reflected by phRAST evidence of allergen-specific IgE antibodies. By intradermal and phRAST testing, these investigators examined 660 adults for sensitivity to three common allergens: cat dander, house dust mite, and grass pollen. Analysis of their discordant results and assay of the sera for the presence of immunoglobulin G (IgG)-4 levels led them to theorize that these antibodies may play a role in the disagreement between test methods. They found that only 18% of patients with contradictory responses to cat-allergy testing had IgG-4 in their blood, and none of the other three test antigens were associated with allergen-specific IgG-4. The authors concluded that IgE levels were too low to be detected.

One of the more recent articles to examine the relationship of *in vitro* to *in vivo* assessment methods was Williams et al (1992), who introduced the use of the receiver-operating characteristic curve to analyze data received from skin tests vs various types of *in vitro* tests. Their studies showed that sensitivity for phRAST ranged from 0.15 to 0.72, and for mRAST from 0.35 to 0.91. Corresponding figures for specificity ranges were 0.90 to 1.0 and 0.79 to 0.95. These results have been questioned and evaluated critically by Nalebuff (presented at the AAOA Annual Meeting, Washington DC, 1992), but the authors correctly point out that skin tests or *in vitro* tests are themselves diagnostic of clinical sensitivity and that "history and clinical judgment remain essential for assessing the significance and relevance of positive and negative test results."

Conclusions

Many studies have compared the skin prick test, the intradermal skin test, and provocation with the RAST, most commonly phRAST. The majority of these studies demonstrate a strong correlation among the modalities. The approach to an initial work-up of a patient with suspected allergies requires consideration of a number of factors that, in combination, help to indicate the appropriate tool for a specific patient. It is important to keep in mind that no test is perfect, and regardless of which is utilized, it is the total accumulation of knowledge about a patient that allows the physician to make an accurate clinical assessment.

References

1. American Academy of Allergy and Immunology. Position statement: The use of *in vitro* tests for IgE antibody in the specific diagnosis of IgE mediated disorders and in the formulation of allergen immunotherapy. *J Allerg Clin Immunol* 1992;90(2):263–267.
2. Kniker W. The choice of allergy skin testing versus *in vitro* determination of specific IgE: No longer as issue? (editorial). *Ann Allergy* 1989;373–374.

3. Stenius B. Skin and provocation tests with *Dermatophagoides pteronyssinus* in allergic rhinitis. Comparison of prick and intracutaneous skin test methods and correlation with specific IgE. *Acta Allergol* 1973;28:81–100.
4. Norman P, Lichtenstein L, Ishizaka K. Diagnostic tests in ragweed hay fever—A comparison of direct skin test, IgE antibody measurements, and basophil histamine release. *J Allerg Clin Immunol* 1973;52(4):210–224.
5. Berg T, Johansson S. Allergy diagnosis with the radioallergosorbent test—A comparison with the results of skin and provocation testing in an unselected group of children with asthma and hay fever. *J Allerg Clin Immunol* 1974;54(4):209–221.
6. Ahlstedt S, Eriksson N, Lindgren S, Roth A. Specific IgE determination by RAST compared with skin and provocation tests in allergy diagnosis with birch pollen, timothy pollen, and dog epithelium allergens. *Clin Allergy* 1974;4:131–140.
7. Perera M, Bernstein I, Michael G, Johansson S. Predictability of the radioallergosorbent test (RAST) in ragweed pollenosis. *Amer Rev Resp Dis* 1975;111:605–610.
8. Bryant D, Burns M, Lazarus L. The correlation between skin test, bronchial provocation tests and serum levels of IgE specific for common allergens in patients with asthma. *Clin Allergy* 1975;5:145–157.
9. Nalebuff D, Fadal R, Ali M. Predictive value of laboratory tests—diagnostic skin test and RAST models. In Fadal R, Nalebuff D, eds. *RAST in Clinical Allergy*, Carlsbad, CA: Symposia Foundation; 1989, pp 165–179.
10. Kraft D, Wide L. Clinical patterns and results of radioallergosorbent test (RAST) and skin tests in penicillin allergy. *Br J Dermatol* 1976;94:593–601.
11. Reddy P, Nagaya H, Pascual H, Lee S, et al. Reappraisal of intracutaneous tests in the diagnosis of reaginic allergy. *J Allerg Clin Immunol* 1978;61(1):36–41.
12. Brown W, Halonen M, Kaltenborn W, Barebee R. The relationship of respiratory allergy, skin test reactivity, and serum IgE in a community population sample. *J Allerg Clin Immunol* 1979;63(5):328–335.
13. Fadal R, Nalebuff D. Allergic skin testing: A clinical evaluation. In Johnson F, ed. *Allergy including IgE in Diagnosis and Treatment*, Chicago: Yearbook Medical Publishers; 1979: 85–93.
14. Vanto T, Viander M, Koivikko A. Skin prick test in the diagnosis of dog dander allergy. *Clin Allergy* 1980;10:121–132.
15. Menardo J, Bousquet J, Michel F. Comparison of three prick test methods with the intradermal test and with the RAST in the diagnosis of mite allergy. *Ann Allergy* 1982;48:235–239.
16. Bousquet J, Lebel B, Dhivert H, Bataille Y, et al. Nasal challenge with pollen grains, skin prick tests and specific IgE in patients with grass pollen allergy. *Clin Allergy* 1987;17:529–536.
17. Huggins K, Brostoff J. Local production of specific IgE antibodies in allergic-rhinitis patients with negative skin tests. *Lancet* 1975; July 26:148–150.
18. Van der Zee J, De Groot H, Van Swieten P, Jansen H, et al. Discrepancies between the skin test and IgE antibody assays: Study of histamine release, complement activation *in vitro*, and occurrence of allergen specific IgE. *J Allerg Clin Immunol* 1988;82:270–281.
19. Williams P, Dolen W, Koepke J, Selner J. Comparison of skin testing and three in vitro assays for specific IgE in the clinical evaluation of immediate hypersensitivity. *Ann Allergy* 1992;68:35–45.

· 5 ·

The Relationship Between SET and In Vitro Testing

RICHARD L. MABRY, M.D., F.A.C.S., F.A.A.O.A.

The Importance of Skin Tests to the Allergist Using In Vitro Methods

In vitro assays for allergen-specific immunoglobulin E (IgE) have captured the attention of patients and medical personnel alike. Despite the obvious advantages of radioallergosorbent test (RAST) and enzyme-linked immunosorbent assay (ELISA) determinations, the physician using them cannot be ignorant of skin testing applications. Immunotherapy based on *in vitro* test results must first be checked by an intracutaneous "vial test,"[1] the interpretation of which demands a knowledge of skin whealing responses. Skin testing may also be helpful in resolving questionable or equivocal *in vitro* results. Skin endpoint titration (SET) allows testing of patients who have come from another city for evaluation, with results available within an hour, with the first immunotherapy dose being provided by the endpoint and confirming wheal application for positive antigens. Finally, SET can be used to test for antigens unavailable (for whatever reason) for *in vitro* assay. A knowledge of the principles and applications of skin endpoint titration will allow the physician engaged in the diagnosis and treatment of inhalant allergy to do so most effectively and safely.[2] Thus, it is not incongruous for a volume devoted to *in vitro* testing to contain basic information about SET.

Skin Whealing Responses

The intradermal injection of approximately 0.01 ml of any solution (saline, diluent, antigen extract) will produce a wheal about 4 mm in diameter, which will enlarge within 10 to 15 minutes by physical spreading of the injected material to a final diameter of 5 mm. "Positive" results to allergy testing involve the production of even larger skin wheals through an allergic reaction between the antigen introduced and allergen-specific immunoglobulin E (IgE) bound to skin mast cells. The release of preformed and newly formed mediators of inflammation (histamine, leukotrienes) results in the classic "wheal and flare" response, causing enlargement of the firm, elevated skin wheal, with a surrounding erythema ("flare"). This reaction begins within two to five minutes of the introduction of the antigen, and should reach its maximum size within about 10 to 15 minutes.[3] (Later wheal enlargement may be due to late-phase and delayed reactions, and has a different significance than the acute reactions discussed here).

Skin whealing responses may be diminished or blunted by such factors as the effect of antihistamines and tricyclic antidepressants, and unusual circumstances, such as recent anaphylaxis. On the other hand, some individuals demonstrate skin hyperreactivity (dermatographia), and produce abnormally large skin wheals merely from the physical trauma of the injection, without antigenic stimulation. For this reason, skin testing is preceded by instructions to the patient to omit antihistamines (36 hours for most antihistamines, three to four weeks for astemizole) and tricyclic antidepressants (two to four days) before testing. In addition, a negative control of diluent and a positive control of histamine are injected, and positive or negative whealing, respectively, to these substances indicates that skin testing at this time would be inaccurate. Factors affecting skin testing are listed in Table 5–1.

Skin Endpoint Titration

Conventional skin testing methods involve the introduction of small amounts of antigen at a single concentration via either a skin prick or intradermal injection, with classification of any resulting wheal and flare as negative or positive (graded 1–4+). The initial work of Hansel and refinement of Rinkel[4] showed the accuracy and advantages of testing with progressively more concentrated antigen solutions, until either no response was noted at the highest concentration practicable, or until progressive positive responses were obtained. Using fivefold antigen dilutions, Rinkel noted that such testing provided highly reproducible results. He termed the antigen concentration at which positive whealing was first noted, and which was followed by further even larger wheals using more concentrated antigens, the "endpoint of reaction." The significance of this "skin endpoint titration" (SET) was that it indicated the strongest concentration of each antigen at which immu-

**Table 5–1   Factors Influencing
Skin Whealing Responses***

1. Volume and potency of antigen
2. Reactivity of skin
   a. dermatographic = augmented
   b. elderly, infants = suppressed
3. Concomitant allergen exposure
   a. inhaled antigen
   b. cross-reactive inhaled antigen
   c. concomitant food
4. Pharmacotherapeutic agents
   a. antihistamines = suppression
   b. tricyclic antidepressants = suppression
5. Blocking antibodies from prior immunotherapy
6. Location on body of testing
   a. back = more sensitive
   b. forearm = less sensitive
7. Axonal reflexes from adjacent tests
8. Time of day

*From Mabry, RL. *Skin Endpoint Titration: History, Theory and Practice*, Meridian Biomedicals, Round Rock, TX, 1992

notherapy could safely be started (even when the antigen in question was in season).

The reader is urged to consult the detailed writings[4–7] available about this technique and avail himself of the numerous courses in its proper application before using it for the first time. However, this brief overview is provided to show the eventual relationship between *in vitro* testing and SET.

Initially, three control wheals are placed: a negative control of diluent (usually phenolated saline), a positive control (histamine diluted to a concentration of 0.004 mg/ml), and a glycerine control (2% glycerine, the concentration of glycerine in the #2 [1:500] antigen dilution, which is normally the most concentrated antigen used in SET). The negative control wheal should be 4 to 6 mm in size at 10 minutes (indicating the absence of skin hyperreactivity), the positive wheal at least 7 mm (indicating an intact wheal and flare response). The size of the glycerine control wheal is noted, and comparison made to wheals of #2 (1:500) antigens in subsequent skin testing. A wheal at this strength should exceed the size of the glycerine control to be considered positive.

After placement of the control wheals, testing with antigens begins. The selection of antigens involves the screening concept popularized by Dr. William King,[8] and it should be possible to initially test with eight to twelve antigens. Positive responses will call for further testing.

The initial injection is with a #6 (1:312,500) concentration. If a wheal of less than 7 mm, not exceeding the diameter of the negative control by 2 mm or more is obtained, then both a #5 (1:62,500) and #4 (1:12,500) concentrations are applied. The reason for applying both is that even if the #5 is positive (diameter exceeds that of the negative control by 2 mm or more), a "confirming wheal" at the next stronger concentration must be placed (which should exceed the diameter of the preceding positive wheal by 2 mm or more). This progressive positive whealing established the first positive wheal as the endpoint. If negative wheals are obtained, the #3 (1:2500) and #2 (1:500) concentrations are tested.

Some clinicians test with #1 (1:100) antigens if the patient's history and circumstances dictate. This may cause problems for the novice, as positive reactions to the glycerine (10% at this concentration) and the inability to check a confirming wheal make decisions to treat at this level difficult.

Certain unusual whealing patterns ("flash" response, "plateau") may occur. The former is a series of negative wheals followed by an extremely large positive wheal, and is normally the result of the recent ingestion of a cross-reacting food. The latter is a titration in which two or more identical initial positive wheals are obtained before wheal size progression occurs. The reader should consult more detailed information on SET for the causes and proper interpretation of these responses.[3,4]

After determination of the endpoint for the screening antigens, and subsequent testing with additional relevant antigens, it is possible to formulate a treatment vial in which each 0.50 ml contains the antigenic equivalent of 0.50 ml of the endpoint concentration for each individual antigen. This is the basic premise of SET-based antigen mixing, and allows dosage which is individualized according to the sensitivity of the patient of each specific antigen. Arithmetically, it is easiest for the novice to grasp the concepts associated with the one-to-one relationship of concentrations of antigen in the test and the treatment vial. The more experienced individual can alter the vial composition and size according to individual preference (making each 0.1 cc of the treatment mix antigenically equivalent to 0.2 cc of the test dose).

More detailed information regarding testing and treatment using SET may be found in the first of the AAOA Monograph Series, *Skin Endpoint Titration.*[7]

Relationship of SET to the F/N Modified RAST

The initial efforts involving *in vitro* testing for allergen-specific IgE were hampered by a scoring system that did not coincide with skin test results. The modification of RAST scoring by Drs. Fadal and Nalebuff[9] (the F/N Modified RAST) not only increased the clinical sensitivity of the test, but the fivefold increments of this scoring system were found to parallel skin test results using the fivefold SET methodology of Rinkel.[4] Because skin tests tend to be slightly more sensitive (or RAST results more specific, depending on one's point of view), RAST generally gives a test score that corresponds to a SET endpoint one class higher (for example, RAST class 3 equivalent to SET endpoint at a #4 concentration). It is important to realize that this correlation has been best established between F/N RAST results and SET (Table 5–2). Although most other *in vitro* testing methods attempt to maintain this relationship, the exact correlation between *in vitro* test results and those obtained by SET must be established by experience for the specific testing modality employed.

Application of SET to In Vitro-Based Immunotherapy

When immunotherapy is based on skin testing, the same antigen stock bottles are used to formulate both the testing and treatment vials. In other words, the testing material and treating material are essentially the same. This is unfortunately not the case in *in vitro*-based diagnosis and treatment. Although the relationship of *in vitro* results to SET has been thoroughly explored, individual variations exist. Therefore, any treatment antigen vial prepared on the basis of *in vitro* tests must be tested on the patient's skin before further injections are given. A number of methods for this "vial testing" exist, and the clinician must adopt the one with which he feels most comfortable. More details on vial testing are found in this book, Chapter X, but a summation of the usual types follows.

The most common method of vial testing is the formulation of a treatment vial prepared from antigens at concentrations one fivefold dilution weaker ("RAST −1") than the RAST score. A skin test with this vial, which yields a wheal of 13 mm or less in diameter indicates that the vial is safe for immunotherapy. It is possible to perform an "incremental vial test"[1] by skin testing every positive antigen determined by RAST testing at a RAST −1 level, then adjusting the concentration of each antigen in the final treatment

Table 5–2   Relationship of SET- and RAST-Based* Immunotherapy

SET ENDPOINT	ANTIGEN CONCENTRATION[†]	RAST 0[‡]	RAST −1[§]
#1	1:100	1:100	1:500
#2	1:500	1:500	1:2500
#3	1:2500	1:2500	1:12,500
#4	1:12,500	1:12,500	1:62,500
#5	1:62,500	1:62,500	1:312,500
#6	1:312,500	1:312,500	1:312,500[¶]

*Also true of many ELISA systems.
[†]Weight/volume, if "concentrate" is 1:20.
[‡]Aggressive regimen, which treats RAST score as endpoint.
[§]Usual regimen, which initiates treatment one class weaker than RAST score.
[¶]Rarely necessary to begin treatment at strengths weaker than #6 dilution.
From Mabry (1992).

Table 5-3   **Technique of Incremental Vial Test Antigen**
at RAST −1 Concentration

WHEAL SIZE	ACTION
<7 mm	Apply stronger concentrations until endpoint determined
7–10 mm	Treat at RAST −1 for this antigen
11–13 mm	Treat at RAST −2 for this antigen
14 mm+	Apply RAST −3 wheal; if acceptable, treat at RAST −3

vial according to the wheals obtained (Table 5-3). Some clinicians determine the correlation between RAST and SET scores by testing volunteers, staff and family, and use this information to make up a treatment vial, which is then vial tested in the usual fashion.[3] If an unacceptable reaction is obtained, this treatment vial is subjected to several fivefold dilutions, SET is done on the vial, and treatment is then initiated at this lower level. This last maneuver may result in the patient receiving a few more injections than using a more aggressive approach, but it has much to recommend it to the novice until more experience is gained. It is obvious that whatever form of vial testing is chosen, a knowledge of normal and abnormal whealing responses is necessary for proper interpretation of the results obtained.

Circumstances may exist in which a patient is receiving immunotherapy based on *in vitro* testing, but it becomes advantageous to test for one or two other antigens and add them to the treatment vial. SET can be quickly and simply accomplished in a single visit, without waiting for the results of *in vitro* testing. It is then possible, using the knowledge of preparing treatment vials based on SET results, to simply add the new antigens to the current treatment vial at the endpoint concentrations, and proceed with immunotherapy. Familiarity with SET principles of testing and treatment will allow the practitioner to move freely between the two modalities, deriving the greatest benefit from each.

Conclusions

In vitro testing methods offer significant advantages over skin testing, even the most efficient skin test methodology, SET. However, the individual administering allergy immunotherapy based on these methods must understand and at times rely on SET for both the safety and benefit of patients receiving this therapy.

References

1. Mabry RL. Blending skin endpoint titration and *in vitro* methods in clinical practice. *Otol Clin No Amer* 1992;25:61–70.

2. King HC. Blending *in vitro* and *in vivo* techniques. In King HC, ed. *An Otolaryngologist's Guide to Allergy.* New York: Thieme Medical Publishers; 1990:97–103.
3. Mabry RL. Skin Endpoint Titration: History, Theory and Practice. Round Rock, TX: Meridian Biomedicals; 1992.
4. Rinkel HJ. The management of clinical allergy (I, II, III). *Arch Otolaryngol* 1962;76:491–508, 1963;77:42–75, and 1963;77:205–225.
5. King WP. The role of the skin end point titration method in allergy. In Goldman JL, ed. *The Principles and Practice of Rhinology.* New York: John Wiley & Sons; 1987:283–292.
6. King HC. Endpoint titration and immunotherapy. *Otol Clin No Amer* 1985;18:703–717.
7. Mabry RL, ed. *Skin Endpoint Titration.* New York: Thieme Medical Publishers; 1992. AAOA Monograph Series.
8. King WP. Efficacy of a screening radioallergosorbent test. *Arch Otolaryngol* 1982;108:781–786.
9. Nalebuff DJ, Fadal RG, Ali M. The study of IgE in the diagnosis of allergic disorders in an otolaryngology practice. *Otolaryngol Head Neck Surg* 1979;87:351–358.

Suggested Additional Reading

AAOA: 1983 Position Statements of the American Academy of Otolaryngic Allergy and Elaboration of Position Statements of the American Academy of Otolaryngic Allergy, Washington, AAOA, 1983.
Council on Scientific Affairs (AMA): *In vivo* diagnostic testing and immunotherapy for allergy. *JAMA* 1987;258:1363–1367.

· 6 ·

In Vitro Assays:
Screening Procedures

WILLIAM P. KING, M.D., F.A.C.S., F.A.A.O.A.

A radioallergosorbent test (RAST) procedure was designed by Wide in 1967[1] shortly after the discovery of IgE in late 1965 by Johansson and Ishizaka. The original commercial RAST procedure, the Phadebas RAST, proved to be unpopular because of the high specificity, which in turn resulted in clinically obvious false-negative responses. This problem was corrected in 1978 with the development of the Fadal-Nalebuff modified RAST.[2] This technique offered the clinician high specificity with satisfactory sensitivity. The physician then had available an in-vitro allergy test that was not only accurate, but also safe and convenient to patient and doctor alike. There remained only one problem and that was, as is so often the case, cost. This deterrent was more an apparition than fact for the positive-responding patient. Allergy-care cost is composed of the sum of expenditures for initial tests, number of injections required to achieve the immunotherapy goal, and morbidity cost, including the cost of medications required to control symptoms. A RAST-tested patient requires far fewer injections to achieve treatment results, with an overall decrease in total cost. Unfortunately, such is not the case for the negative-responding patient. For the latter, skin testing to identify nonatopy is less expensive than a full RAST battery. Thus, the dilemma, and, thus, the motive for the development of an efficacious RAST screen to cost-efficiently identify the nonatopic patient.

Screening Procedures

Total IgE

The paper radioimmunosorbent assay test (PRIST) for the identification of the serum total IgE was developed before the RAST. It was hoped that the test would serve as a cost-effective *in vitro* screen for nonatopy. More or less empirically, a total IgE score of 100 U/ml or less was thought to essentially rule out the presence of any significant patient atopy, while scores of 100 U/ml or more indicated a very high likelihood of an existing atopic problem. Unfortunately, while total IgE may be utilized as a rough guide for the likelihood of atopy, it has been found unreliable as a definitive screening test. In some patients with apparently high nonspecific IgE serum content, specific biological inhalant IgE tests have been negative in the face of a total IgE score above 400 U/ml, while others with a total score below 10 U/ml still present a class IV or V specific biological inhalant count.

To illustrate, in a 1982 retrospective study of 100 consecutive allergy patients seen in the author's office, their total IgE results were compared with those of their specific IgE in 16 to 20 antigen RAST batteries.[3] The patients chosen presented a wide variety of complaints, including allergic rhinitis, chronic rhinosinusitis, asthma, urticaria and angioedema, frequent respiratory tract infections, recurrent acute and chronic laryngitis, persistent or recurrent serous otitis media, and severe recurrent vascular headaches. As would be expected, the higher the total IgE count, the more likelihood of positive specific response in the full battery (Table 6–1). It should be noted, however, that in those 44 patients exhibiting a total IgE of between 11 U/ml and 200 U/ml, only 50% proved to have a positive responder on the full battery, and, when the total IgE score was 10 U/ml or below, 33% (3 out of 9 patients) still had at least one positive responder. One of these three had a perhaps equivocal class I response, a second one a more significant class II response, and the third certainly a very significant class III response.

Likewise, Nalebuff[4] reports that "while those persons classified as 'positive atopics' were found to have significantly higher geometric mean levels of total IgE than the others, the ranges of these levels within each of the three groups were so wide that they could not adequately serve to identify an individual atopic patient." In the same paper he reported a similar study of 100 consecutive patients, where the total IgE of eight nonatopic patients ranged between

Table 6–1   Reliance of Total IgE Screen in 100 Cases

U/ml	FULL BATTERY POSITIVES	# OF CASES
401–683	99%	30 of 31
201–400	81%	13 of 16
11–200	50%	22 of 44
0–10	33%	3 of 9

4 and 440 U/ml, with a geometric mean of 30 U/ml. Fourteen equivocal atopic patients, that is, patients with only class I positive specific responses, ranged between 8 and 340 U/ml with a geometric mean of 90 U/ml. The remaining 78 positive atopic patients, that is, those with a class II or above specific antigen response, ranged between 8 and 900 U/ml, with a geometric mean of 290 U/ml. Hamburger[5] also spoke of the genetic implications of observed positive RASTs in low IgE individuals.

One may then ask, is a total IgE of any clinical value? As stated, it does serve as a rough guide to the likelihood of the presence of IgE-mediated allergy, but it is certainly not absolute. It may also serve in infants as a prognosticator of atopy to come, allowing preventive action through environmental control and preventive food allergy diet. Lastly, total IgE may also serve as an aid to interpretation of a borderline positive or negative result. In summary, total IgE test procedures are not cost effective as a single test screen for atopy.

Screening RAST

The "Representative" Approach

In the previously mentioned author's study[3] of 100 consecutive office allergy patients, on their total of 16 to 20 antigen RAST battery, 31% proved totally negative, while 69% proved positive to at least one allergen. Of the latter, there was only one positive allergen responder in 12 of the patients, and two in five other patients. In these 17%, the positive-responding allergens were almost invariably either house dust mites, or epidermals, showing that these common household antigens are frequently solitary but often severe offenders and cannot be effectively screened.

The high percentage of negative responders struck a sympathetic note in the ever loudening cry for medical cost containment. There was observed a significant tendency for the occurrence of multiple sensitivities when application of the Kendall rank correlation procedure revealed a high probability rate for mutual positive responses between all tested allergens.[6]

In consideration of this study's observations, a screening RAST battery[3] was devised consisting of house dust mite farinae, two molds, Alternaria and the highly Kendall rank correlating Mucor; three pollens, each representing the apparent prominent area pollen for each of the tree; grass and weed groups, specifically, mountain cedar, Bermuda grass, and short ragweed. Lastly, in view of the previously presented statistics, any epidermals to which the patient was significantly exposed by history were also included. A retrospective study was then accomplished by applying this empirically created screening RAST battery to the results of 469 previously accomplished full RAST batteries. If one considered the previously stated percentage of 30% negative responders, this retrospective study would total 670 patients.

The positive-responding patients were subdivided into two groups of responders, the first or "exact" group included class I equivocal responders, while the second "definite" group contained only class II and above responders. Utilizing the standard formulas for test efficiency and test sensitivity (test efficiency = true-positive + true-negative/grand total × 100, and test sensitivity = true-positive/true-positive + false-negative × 100),[7] the impressive figures indicated in Table 6–2 for the screening RAST were deduced. Curiosity then demanded further evaluation of the efficacy of the separate mold and pollen prognosticators as screens for their respective groups. These mini-screens were also calculated as reported in Table 6–2. The results were remarkable in all categories, with the small caveat in the pollen "exact" category, where it is obvious that some class I responders will be missed utilizing this screen.

As advised by the author[3] for a fine tuning of all geographic area screens, an allergen prevalence evaluation for the Corpus Christi, Texas area was then accomplished, resulting in the utilization of Cladosporium mold rather than Mucor, and oak tree replacing mountain cedar on the screen battery. The American Academy of Otolaryngic Allergy advises routine utilization of such a screening RAST prior to the accomplishment of further RAST testing in consideration of its medically efficacious cost containment virtues.[8]

Two additional perennial antigens, when available for testing, were later added to the recommended screening RAST: cockroach and house dust mite pteronyssinus. The screening RAST thus contains all of the household perennials present in the full battery.

Before April 1986, only five airborne molds were commercially available for RAST testing. At that time, Pharmacia made available 10 additional airborne molds (Table 6–3). This prompted a study[9] concerning the efficacy of the then recommended two-mold Alternaria/Cladosporium mold screen for the now possible 15-mold battery. Five of these ten molds were commonly found in the Corpus Christi area. When these five new molds were added to the five old molds previously tested, 83 positive mold responders were identified in 275 patients. Interestingly, one of these five new molds, Helminthosporium, was found to be the second most common positive mold responder, after Alter-

Table 6–2 Screening RAST Efficiency and Sensitivity

	EFFICIENCY		SENSITIVITY	
	*Exact (%)**	*Definite (%)*	*Exact (%)*	*Definite (%)*
Screening RAST	96.0	99.4	94.2	99.2
Pollen mini-screen	88.0	98.7	78.1	97.6
Mold mini-screen	96.9	99.7	91.5	99.2

*Exact, includes equivocal Class I responders. Definite, includes only Class II or higher responders.

Table 6–3   Airborne Mold Available Battery

OLD	NEW
Alternaria alternata	*Helminthosporium halodes**
Aspergillus fumigatus	*Curvularia lunata**
Cladosporium herbarum	*Fusarium moniliforme**
Mucor racemosus	*Epicoccum purpurascens**
Penicillium natatum	*Stemphylium botryosum**
	Aureobasidium pullulans
	Botrytis cinerea
	Phoma betae
	Rhizopus nigricans
	Trichoderma viride

*Five new molds commonly present in Corpus Christi area

naria. Three variations of mold screens were retrospectively evaluated for the efficiency and sensitivity. When the Alternaria/Cladosporium screen was evaluated, eight class I positive responses and five class II or higher missed responses were found. The next most efficient screen was Alternaria/ Helminthosporium, where, again, there were eight class I positives, but only two class II or higher missed responses. The most efficient was a combination of Alternaria/Cladosporium/Helminthosporium, where there were only five class I missed responses. When the formulas for efficiency and sensitivity were again applied, the efficiency in the "exact" group was 98.7% and the "definite" group was 100%. The sensitivity in the "exact" group was 94% and in the "definite" group 100%.

The current screening RAST now utilized in this office consists of nine allergens plus PRN epidermals, as listed in Table 6–4.

Considering the previously noted 30% full RAST battery negativity on suspected allergy patients, plus the near 20% where the positive responses were limited to household perennials, the screening RAST as recommended

Table 6–4   Screening RAST

Household perennials	House dust mite farinae
	House dust mite pteronyssinus
	Cockroach
	P.R.N. epidermal
Molds	Alternaria
	Cladosporium
	Helminthosporium
Pollens	Rye grass
	Oak tree
	Short ragweed

should suffice for almost 50% of all tested patients. Also, when more testing is indicated because of positive responses to either the tested molds or pollens, testing in only one of these categories may be necessary, again resulting in cost containment.

Numerical Approach

Nalebuff[4] also advocated the use of a screening RAST, basing his testimonial on a mathematical-percentage approach. He noted that the prevalence of sensitization to antigens with high allergenicity varied widely, ranging from 20 to 80%. He proposed a six-antigen screening RAST battery, including June grass, short ragweed, house dust mite, Alternaria, oak tree, and animal dander. He mathematically illustrated how only 3% of true atopic patients should be negative to a five-antigen screening panel if one assumed the probability of each antigen for positivity is only 50%. In actuality, he states, less than 1% of atopic patients are negative to such a screening panel because the prevalence is 80% to June grass and 65% to ragweed in atopic patients.

Utilizing his six-antigen screen as outlined for consideration retrospectively on 100 consecutive rhinitis patients, all 78 of the positive atopic patients and 12 of 14 equivocal atopic patients, that is, those patients with only class I responders, would have been detected for an overall sensitivity level of 98%. Note that, even though his patients were limited to those with rhinitis complaints, he still had a 22% negativity rate, not dissimilar from the previously mentioned overall 30% when patients with allergy complaints other than rhinitis were included.

New Generation

After the original screening RAST was suggested in 1982, a proliferation of screens were placed on the commercial market. Like all allergy tests, the screens may be categorized as quantitative or qualitative. Quantitative tests not only tell if the patient is atopic, but also provide information on degree of sensitivity to each allergen in its particular screening battery, for example, the King and Nalebuff suggested screening RASTs. All of these newly presented screens are purely qualitative; that is, they report merely if the patient is atopic or not. Once the "atopic" diagnosis is made, individual tests must then be done on each included antigen to determine which of the antigens are positive responders to what degree they are positive for consideration of the staring dosage for immunotherapy. The first such qualitative tests offered comprised multiple allergens on a single RAST disc. In actuality, this concept was originally introduced by Merrett and Merrett in 1978,[10] when they utilized a RAST screen of three allergens coupled on a single solid-phase cellulosupport disc. On recheck of the specific allergens, house dust mite, grass, and cat dander, this single-disc screen proved to be 97% sensitive and 100% specific.

In 1983, a so-called horizontal RAST screen was offered by Pharmacia[4] that provided a number of area grass mixes on one disc, along with similar area tree mixes, area weed mixes, a mold mix, a house dust mite mix, and an animal dander mix. Utilizing these mixes, a total screen across the board could be accomplished with six RAST tests. In 1984, a so-called vertical RAST screen was offered by Ventrex,[4] placing June and Bermuda grass, short ragweed, English plantain, oak, and elm on one disc and Alternaria and house dust mite farinae on a second disc. This variety of a two-disc screen somewhat imitated the original suggested screening RAST. Once again, these tests are purely qualitative and, if a positive response results, one must go back and test each contained antigen separately to ascertain specific positivity and degree of sensitivity. Clearly, for the positive-responding patient, such qualitative screens are not cost-effective.

In the ensuing years, a number of inventive and ingenious screening tests have been placed on the market. One provides the simplicity of a dip-stick test, others provide a syringe barrel device or liquid antigen for simplified testing. Others, I am sure, shall be forthcoming. It must be emphasized, however, that all of these tests are qualitative, that is, provide only a simple "yes" or "no."

Conclusions

The American Academy of Otolaryngic Allergy,[8] in my view, rightfully recommends the use of some form of screening procedure prior to continuation of full inhalant allergy testing, whether by *in vitro* or skin technique.

Thus, the final decision is not whether to use a screen, but which variety. The author suggests the following: that qualitative screens be used by the nonallergist to confirm suspicion of atopy for appropriate referral, or for the allergy specialist to cost-effectively confirm a suspicion of nonatopy. It is further recommended that the quantitative screens be used by allergy specialists to confirm cost-effectively suspicion of atopy, and to appropriately limit the number of tests accomplished.

References

1. Wide L, Bennich H, Johansson SGO. Diagnosis of allergy by *in vitro* test for allergen antibodies. *Lancet* 1967;2:1105.
2. Nalebuff DJ. Study of IgE In The Diagnosis and Management of Allergy. Transactions American Society of Ophthalmology and Otolaryngology. *Allergy* 1978;18:60.
3. King WP. Efficacy of a screening radioallergosorbent test. *Arch Otolaryngology* 1982;781–786.
4. Nalebuff DJ. Use of RAST screening in clinical allergy; a cost-effective approach to patient care. *Ear, Nose, Throat* 1985; March:107–121.

5. Hamburger RN. The genetic implications of positive RAST in low IgE individuals. *Immunol Allergy Pract* 1980;2:8–12.
6. Alder HL, Roessler E. *Introduction to Probability and Statistics*, 6th ed. San Francisco: W. H. Freeman and Co., 1977.
7. Galen RS, Gambino SR, eds. *Beyond Normality: The Predictive Value and Efficiency of Medical Diagnosis*. New York: John Wiley and Sons, Inc., 1975;13, 33.
8. Position Statement of The American Academy of Otolaryngologic Allergy, Washington, D.C., 1989.
9. King WP. Clinical significance of molds newly available for radioallergosorbent testing. *Arch Otolaryngology* 1989;101:1–4.
10. Merrett J, Merrett TG. RAST atopy screen. *Clinical Allergy* 1978;8:235–240.

7

Selection of Initial Immunotherapy Doses Based on the Modified RAST Result

DONALD J. NALEBUFF, M.D.
BARBARA CORDES, R.N.

For more than 80 years allergen immunotherapy has been an important cornerstone in the management of allergic rhinitis and still remains the only specific treatment available with the potential for cure. Successful immunotherapy has been documented in treatment-resistant patients suffering from allergic rhinitis due to ragweed, grass, mountain cedar and birch pollen, house-dust mite, and cat dander sensitivity.[1-7]

Specific clinical situations where its application is appropriate include patients who respond inadequately to environmental control, who experience insufficient relief or unpleasant side-effects from pharmacotherapy, patients having symptoms that extend over two or more seasons, patients who have symptoms that become progressively worse each year and their severity is more of a problem than the inconvenience and costs involved with immunotherapy. An important final consideration is whether the patient is likely to comply with the schedule of injections for a duration of several years.

In several controlled studies[8-16] confirming the efficacy of allergen immunotherapy the following conclusions are indisputable: (1) It has been found effective only in immunoglobulin E (IgE)-mediated disease. (2) The results of therapy are specific; that is, the patients experience relief only for those administered allergens, meaning symptoms due to other allergens do not change during therapy. (3) The administration of high-doses (maximum tolerated dose) of allergenically active material is required to produce the immunologic changes observed in clinically improved patients. A limiting factor in achieving such effective dosage, however, has been the threat of causing undesirable systemic reactions. It has been reported that these reactions occur at a greater frequency and severity in those patients with high serum levels of allergen-specific IgE as measured by the P-K transfer technique. In addition, an inverse relationship has been found to exist between the highest tolerated dose and this serum antibody titer.[17,18]

Since 1967, with the development of the radioallergosorbent (RAST) test, physicians now have available a simple test for the detection of this antibody in serum and the *in vitro* estimation of these titers without any of the problems inherent in performing P-K titers.[19] The role of RAST in predicting individual dose tolerance was first investigated by Bernstein in 1975 in forty ragweed sensitive patients.[20] They participated in a rapid desensitization experiment in which allergen doses were progressively increased and administered every 30 minutes to the point of maximum tolerance determined by the size of local reaction at the site of injections or mild systemic symptoms. It was observed that patients with high RAST scores could tolerate only small doses of allergen and developed reactions more readily. As a result, Bernstein advised that such patients be routinely started with extremely dilute material and that doses be raised cautiously.

These observations suggested to us that individual sensitivity to clinically-relevant allergens as determined by the Modified RAST (mRAST) procedure could be used as a guide in selecting safe initial dose levels.[21] We have found that by employing this methodology untoward reactions are essentially avoidable. In addition, by incorporating the direct measurement of specific-IgE antibody into the decision making, allergen immunotherapy treatment is limited to those patients with detectable levels of serum specific IgE antibody. The net effect of incorporating the direct measurement of specific-IgE antibody into the decision making process has been that: (1) fewer patients are started on immunotherapy, (2) initial treatment doses for allergens associated with low mRAST scores are administered at higher levels than previously considered possible, and (3) physicians are alerted to those situations in which the patient is at risk for having an adverse reaction.

Technique of mRAST-Based Immunotherapy

In mRAST-based immunotherapy the recommended initial doses are given at concentrations as listed in Table 7–1. When more than one allergen is mixed in a treatment vial, the various strengths are adjusted to be in inverse propor-

Table 7–1   Concentration of Initial Doses
Based on the Modified RAST Score

| CLASS | COUNTS | ALLERGEN CONCENTRATION (w/v)* | |
		RAST −1	*RAST 0*
0	250–500		
1/0	501–750	1:500	1:100
1	751–1600	1:500	1:100
2	1601–3600	1:2500	1:500
3	3601–8000	1:12,500	1:2500
4	8001–18,000	1:62,500	1:12,500
5	18,001–40,000	1:312,500	1:62,500

*The RAST −1 allergen concentration is the recommended initial dose level in RAST-based immunotherapy. Allergens with equivocal scores are included in the treatment set when judged to be clinically relevant.

tion to each individual serum antibody concentration. Our patients are regularly started at allergen concentrations of 1:500 w/v for those allergens with low serum specific IgE levels (mRAST class 1 scores). As the serum antibody concentration rises, the suggested initial dose is proportionally decreased in fivefold increments. For those allergens in which the specific antibody score is extremely high (mRAST class 5 scores) the recommended initial doses is significantly lower at an allergen concentration of 1:312,500 w/v. This range of initial doses has been characterized as a RAST −1 dose. In our experience, attempts to be more conservative by starting patients at dose levels below this (RAST −2) increases the level of the patient sensitivity and makes the subsequent raising of the doses more difficult.

Before staring such immunotherapy, however, it is mandatory that a small amount of the incriminated allergens in the treatment vial be placed intradermally as a skin-test challenge (enough of the allergen must be injected to produce a 4 mm skin weal). This step is done to insure that there has not been a laboratory error in either the test performance or in the formulation of the treatment vials. The patient is then observed and if in ten minutes this *in vivo* challenge produces a weal of 15 mm or less, the recommended dose can be safely given subcutaneously. While this challenge is performed in all patients, it is especially important for class 1 through class 3 allergens, where the suggested mRAST based doses are high (1:500 to 12,500 w/v). With class four and five allergens, the *in vivo* challenges are less important because the suggested doses (1:62,500 to 1:312,500 w/v) are consistent with levels considered safe, even for extremely sensitive patients. Nevertheless, even in these situations, the *in vivo* challenge serves the useful purpose of confirming the biological potency of the highly diluted allergen extract. Only rarely, in our practice, have the skin test challenge responses suggested that the mRAST-based dose would be excessive.

After the initial doses have been administered and tolerated, injections are raised at subsequent visits (unless the clinical response suggests it would not be safe) until the dose reaches maximum tolerated levels. Doses are incrementally raised from 0.05 ml to 0.5 ml (Table 7–2). Once these have been tolerated, a new treatment set is made at the next highest concentration and the escalation continued as described in Figure 7–1.

Preparation of Serially-Diluted Stock Solutions

We use 50% glycerinated allergen extracts because these maintain potency well; these are obtained at a 1:20 w/v concentration in the 30 ml vial size. To insure a constant rotation of fresh solutions, we work with small amounts of solution in both the stock and treatment vials (2.5 ml). Five stock solutions are prepared for each potentially incriminating allergen as follows: 2.5 ml of the 1:20 w/v concentrated extracts is withdrawn from the large vials (30.0 ml) and placed into an empty, sterile 2.5 ml vial for subsequent use in the stock vial trays. Fivefold stock dilutions of this material are then prepared from the 1:20 w/v stock concentrate vials. Preparation of stock dilutions D/1 (1:100 w/v) are made from the stock concentrates as follows: 0.5 ml of the 1:20 w/v concentrate plus 2.0 ml phenolated saline diluent will make stock dilution D/1 and give a total volume of 2.5 ml. Preparations of stock dilutions D/2 (1:500 w/v) are made from the D/1 stock dilutions as follows: 0.5 ml of the 1:100 w/v concentration plus 2.0 ml phenolated saline diluent will make stock dilution D/2 and give a total volume of 2.5 ml. Preparation of stock dilutions D/3 (1:2500 w/v) are made from the D/2 stock dilutions as follows: 0.5 ml of the 1:500 w/v concentration plus 2.0 ml phenolated saline diluent will make stock

Table 7–2   Theoretical Treatment Schedule*

INJECTION #	VOLUME (ml)	ROUTE
1	0.02	Intradermal
2	0.05	Subcutaneous
3	0.10	Subcutaneous
4	0.20	Subcutaneous
5	0.30	Subcutaneous
6	0.40	Subcutaneous
7	0.50	Subcutaneous

*Prior to giving the first dose subcutaneously, an intradermal challenge is given (the vial test) to insure that the patient can safely tolerate the selected dose. If the resultant wheal is less than 15 mm, subsequent injections are given subcutaneously as described. Once a dose of 0.5 ml is given and tolerated, a new treatment vial is created at the next five-fold stronger concentration (Fig. 1).

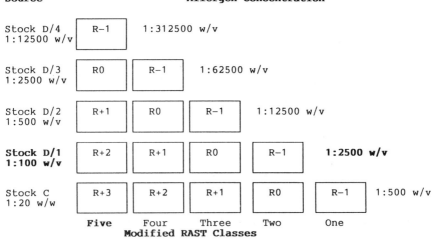

Figure 7–1.   Each allergen is diluted 25× (either by other allergens or diluent) to obtain the proper concentration. For example, a RAST +2 dose of a Class 5 allergen is made from the Stock D/1 (1:100 w/v) and the final concentration is 1:2500 w/v. All class 1–3 allergens will be able to tolerate doses of 1:500 w/v or greater. Proceed with caution with class 4–5 allergens. Immunotherapy doses are escalated to the highest tolerated level. However, raising doses above the RAST +2 level will significantly increase the incidence of systemic reactions.

dilutions D/3 and give a total volume of 2.5 ml. Finally, preparation of stock dilution D/4 (1:12,500 w/v) are made from the D/3 stock dilutions in a similar fashion: 0.5 ml of the 1:2500 w/v concentration plus 2.0 ml phenolated saline diluent will make stock dilution D/4 and give a total volume of 2.5 ml. These five properly labeled stock solutions are used to create individualized treatment sets for our atopic patients (Table 7–3). If one elects to use 5.0 ml vials, one need simply double the values just described.

Table 7–3   RAST Therapy*

NUMBERS	LABEL	CONCENTRATION
1.	Concentrate	1:20 w/v
2.	Stock Dilution #1	1:100 w/v
3.	Stock Dilution #2	1:500 w/v
4.	Stock Dilution #3	1:2500 w/v
5.	Stock Dilution #4	1:12500 w/v

*In RAST-based therapy only five stock vials are required for each allergen. 25-fold dilutions will provide the range of doses needed to create appropriate treatment set vials (1:500 w/v to 1:312,500 w/v).

Preparation of Individual Patient Treatment Vials

The mRAST scores of a typical patient with perennial allergic rhinitis are listed in Figure 7–2. As in this example, there are often varying degrees of sensitivity to individual allergens. Therefore, we recommend that mRAST classes 1, 2, and 3 be placed in one treatment vial (low-level scores) and mRAST class 4 and 5 kept together in a separate treatment vial (high-level scores). A treatment set for this patient is made by taking 0.1 ml from the appropriate stock vial for each clinically-relevant allergen to be included and adding enough phenolated saline diluent to a total volume of 2.5 ml. Each allergen is diluted 25×. One would take 0.2 ml from the appropriate stock vial if 5.0 ml vials are used; thus, a maximum of 25 allergens can be included in a single treatment vial. Once the treatment sets are made up, initial treatment dosages are escalated as described in Table 7–2.

Preparation Of Initial Immunotherapy Treatment Vials Based On The Modified RAST Results In A Typical Atopic Patient

	Counts	(Class)		Counts	(Class)		Counts	(Class)
June Grass	18343	(5)	Maple Tree	1322	(1)	Alternaria	1666	(2)
Bermuda Grass	1200	(1)	**Oak Tree**	9215	**(4)**	Mucor	875	(1)
Timothy Grass	11133	(4)	Elm Tree	4322	(3)	Penicillium	2443	(2)
Short Ragweed	23400	(5)	Birch Tree	344	(0)	Cladosporium	356	(0)
English Plantain	432	(0)	Sycamore Tree	455	(0)	Aspergillus	1423	(1)
Mugwort	254	(0)	White Ash Tree	366	(0)	D. Farinae	370	(0)
Lamb's Quarter	878	(1)	Cat Epithelium	------		D. Pteronyssinus	433	(0)
Dandelion	1143	(1)	Dog Epithelium	------		Cockroach	------	

Volume		Stock Tray (RAST -1 doses)		Dose Concentration
0.1	Bermuda Stock	Concentrate	(1:20 w/v)	1:500 w/v
0.1	Lamb's Quarter	Concentrate	(1:20 w/v)	1:500 w/v
0.1	Dandelion	Concentrate	(1:20 w/v)	1:500 w/v
0.1	Maple Tree	Concentrate	(1:20 w/v)	1:500 w/v
0.1	Mucor	Concentrate	(1:20 w/v)	1:500 w/v
0.1	Aspergillus	Concentrate	(1:20 w/v)	1:500 w/v
0.1	Alternaria	Stock D/1	(1:100 w/v)	1:2500 w/v
0.1	Penicillium	Stock D/1	(1:100 w/v)	1:2500 w/v
0.1	Elm Tree	Stock D/2	(1:500 w/v)	1:12500 w/v

add 1.6 ml Diluent to create a 2.5 ml
Treatment Vial A (Low Sensitivity)

0.1	Oak Tree	Stock D/3	(1:2500 w/v)	1:62500 w/v
0.1	Timothy Grass	Stock D/3	(1:2500 w/v)	1:62500 w/v
0.1	June Grass	Stock D/4	(1:12500 w/v)	1:312500 w/v
0.1	Short Ragweed	Stock D/4	(1:12500 w/v)	1:312500 w/v

add 2.1 ml Diluent to create a 2.5 ml
Treatment Vial B (High Sensitivity)

Figure 7–2. This patient has detectable levels of specific IgE to 13 of the allergies tested by modified RAST. They are separated into two treatment vials so that a more deliberate pace of advance is available for those allergens capable of causing reaction as doses are escalated. These treatment vials are created at the RAST −1 dose level and escalated as shown in Table 7–2.

Results of mRAST-Based Immunotherapy

A review of the mRAST records of patients treated in our clinic reveals that on an average they are sensitive to ten test allergens. Eighty % of the positive scores are at the lower levels (mRAST classes 1–3) (Table 7–4). These allergens are unlikely to cause a constitutional reaction in therapy despite the high initial doses employed. All of our patients have tolerated the initial high doses of these allergens. In these same patients, the remaining twenty percent of incriminated allergens were associated with high levels of specific IgE antibody (mRAST class 4–5 scores) and were started in therapy at the lower dose concentrations. These allergens are also advanced on a more deliberate schedule. They commonly cause large local and even mild constitutional reactions when high dosage levels are attempted. During the past 15 years, the only severe constitutional reactions requiring medical intervention have occurred with those allergens associated with high mRAST scores. In these cases we attempted to raise the dose to levels comparable to those readily obtained by allergens associated with low levels of specific IgE antibody. Once maintenance doses are achieved the interval between injections is widened to a once-a-month schedule.

In a previously published paper on the effects of mRAST-based immunotherapy in 46 allergic rhinitis patients in whom pharmacological agents had failed to provide relief, it was noted that 41/46 patients obtained symptomatic improvement within 24 weeks.[22] In another study, 200 ragweed-sensitive hay-fever patients were also started on treatment with initial doses suggested by their mRAST score.[23] These patients all had positive histories of seasonal rhinitis, occurring from August through October, demonstrated skin reactivity of 3+ or more with a short ragweed extract and a positive nasal or conjunctival provocation on sequential challenge with the ragweed pollen extract at a concentration of 1:100 w/v or less. Ninety serums were scored as mRAST class one for the ragweed allergen and these patients were given high doses of the extract. To stress the system, the doses employed were one fivefold level more concentrated then regularly used. These patients were

Table 7–4   Distribution Of Initial Immunotherapy Doses

MRT CLASS	PERCENTAGE	DOSE SCHEDULE (w/v)*
0	35	—
0/1	5	1:500
1	25	1:500
2	14	1:2,500
3	9	1:12,500
4	7	1:62,500
5	5	1:312,500

*Almost 80% of the initial immunotherapy doses administered were at levels of 1:12500 w/v or greater.

given, as their initial dose, 0.1 ml of a 1:100 w/v material containing 3 µg of Antigen E (AgE); no systemic reactions occurred. One-third of these patients did experience large local reactions, which was attributed to the high concentration of glycerin in the extract at the selected concentration. Fifty-two patients were started on therapy with allergen material at a 1:500 w/v concentration. Only six patients were started at the lowest dose used in this particular study, a concentration of 1:62,500 w/v. Although 70% of these patients (140/200) received 3 µg doses of IgE within the first week of treatment, no constitutional reactions occurred in the entire group.

Similar findings were reported by Young (1981) in a study to determine whether the mRAST score could safely predict a safe initial starting dose.[24] His study included forty patients with a history of rhinitis with a seasonal exacerbation to either timothy or ragweed pollen. All patients had a 2+ or greater skin reaction to the study antigens. Twenty-six of these patients had mRAST class one through three scores and were given the suggested high doses. Fourteen patients were started at a modest dose because of the higher serum antibody levels; all patients were able to tolerate the initial dose without reaction. In a study reported by Santrach (1981), 50 patients were started on immunotherapy with initial doses based on the mRAST score. All 35 patients with class one to class three scores were given their initial doses according to the more aggressive dose schedule (1:100 to 1:2500 w/v) and tolerated the dose without incident. The initial doses were withheld in 15 other patients because the preliminary skin test challenge gave greater than a 15 mm weal. As a result, these investigators reported that thirty-percent (15/50) of their patients could not tolerate the suggested mRAST dose. Examination of the data from these patients shows that the recommended doses were at a 1:312,500 w/v concentration—a level considered safe by most allergists even for their highly sensitive patients. In fact, Santrach and colleagues even noted that the initial doses in the mRAST-based system for such patients are actually less than that recommended by most traditional allergists for such patients.[25] It is likely, therefore, that those patients who did not pass the skin test challenge could have tolerated the suggested initial dose.

In a more recent study comparing the immunologic effects obtained with immunotherapy based on traditional approaches, skin-endpoint titration and RAST-based therapy, Trevino noted that the highest levels of IgG blocking antibody were obtained by the latter technique.[26]

Length of Treatment and Prognosis

The response to immunotherapy remains unpredictable in any given patient. Usually therapy is continued through two or three years of reduced or symptom-free seasons. It is also evident that few patients receive enough benefit from this modality to enable them to discontinue all medication.

While for some patients there is a long-lasting relief, permanent "cure" is rare; it has frequently been observed that relapses occur once therapy has discontinued and such patients may require a repeat course of immunotherapy. Immunotherapy should be discontinued, however, if after two years of uninterrupted maintenance dosage the patient shows no clinical improvement. If the patient has not responded by then, it is unlikely that they will do so should immunotherapy be continued. The measurement of specific IgG antibody should be helpful in deciding the course to be followed in such patients. One must be sure, in those not responding, that other forms of rhinitis are not coexisting and that any physical factors contributing to symptoms, such as septal deviations and turbinate enlargements, are corrected. Some of the causes of immunotherapy failure are listed in Table 7–5.

Conclusions

The net effect of incorporating the direct measurement of specific-IgE antibody into the decision-making in allergy practice has been that fewer patients are started on immunotherapy. High mRAST scores alert the clinician to those situations where specific-IgE antibodies are present at a high enough concentration to cause systemic reactions. Low mRAST scores, on the other hand, allow the physician to be more aggressive both in initiating and advancing the immunotherapy dosages. Limiting this form of therapy to symptomatic patients with measurable levels of specific IgE antibody and the early administration of dose levels known to stimulate the immune system affords the treating physician with a modality which brings science to an area of medical practice that in the past has often functioned more like an art form.

Allergen immunotherapy has a definite role in the overall management of allergic patients. At this point it should be emphasized, however, that the detection of allergen specific IgE levels by the mRAST or other in-vitro methods is not in itself a valid indication for starting patients on immunotherapy. The selection of patients to be started on immunotherapy and the

Table 7–5   Potential Causes of Immunotherapy Failure

1. An incorrect diagnosis was made (a marginal history "confirmed" by a false-positive diagnostic test).
2. Environmental control measures were inadequate.
3. Either the initial selection of clinically relevant antigens was incorrect or additional allergens not included in treatment are present (e.g., new pets).
4. Maintenance doses may not have been high enough to evoke an immune response.
5. Underlying medical problems such as nasal polyps, a deviated nasal septum, or hypothyroidism were missed. The patient uses medications that cause nasal congestion (e.g., reserpine and oral contraceptives).
6. There was an unrecognized concomitant food or chemical intolerance.
7. Poor patient compliance with schedule of therapy injections.

doses finally reached must be made in accordance with the physicians clinical judgment.

References

1. Noon L. Prophylactic inoculation for hay fever. *Lancet* 1911;1:1572.
2. Cooke RA. The treatment of hay fever by active immunization. *Laryngoscope* 1915;25:108.
3. Frankland AW, Augustin R. Prophylaxis of summer hay fever and asthma: A controlled trial comparing crude grass-pollen extracts with the isolated main protein component. *Lancet* 1954;1:1055.
4. Lowell FC, Franklin W. A double-blind study of the effectiveness and specificity of injection therapy in ragweed hayfever. *N Engl J Med* 1965;273:675.
5. Gabriel MHK, et al. Study of prolonged hyposensitization with D. pteronyssinus extract in allergic rhinitis. *Clin Allergy* 1977;7:325.
6. Taylor WW, Ohman JL, Lowell FC. Immunotherapy in cat induced asthma. A double-blind trial with evaluation of bronchial responses to cat allergen and histamine. *J Allergy Clin Immunol* 1978;61:283.
7. Lee LK, Kniker WT, Campos T. Aggressive Coseasonal Immunotherapy in Mountain Cedar Pollen Allergy. *Arch Otolaryngol* 1982;108:787–794.
8. Sherman WB. Changes in serologic reactions and tissue sensitity in hayfever patients during the early months of treatment. *J Immunol* 1941;40:289.
9. Johnstone DE. Study of the role of antigen dose in the treatment of pollenosis and pollen asthma. *J Dis Child* 1957;94:1.
10. Levy DA, et al. Immunologic and cellular changes accompanying the therapy of a pollen allergy. *J Clin Invest* 1971;50:360.
11. Irons JS, Pruzansky JJ, Patterson R. Immunotherapy: mechanisms of action suggested by measurements of immunologic and cellular parameters; allergy grand rounds. *J Allergy Clin Immunol* 1975;56:64.
12. Rocklin RE. Clinical and immunologic aspects of allergen specific immunotherapy in patients with seasonal allergic rhinitis and/or allergic asthma. *J Allergy Clin Immunol* 1983;72:323.
13. Creticos PS. Immunotherapy with allergens. *JAMA* 1992;268:2835–2839.
14. Van Metre TE, Adkinson NF, Lichtenstein LM, et al. A controlled study of the effectiveness of the Rinkel method of immunotherapy for ragweed pollen hay fever. *J Allergy Clin Immunol* 1980;65:288.
15. Van Arsdel PP, Sherman WB. The risk of inducing constitutional reactions in allergic patients. *J Allergy* 1957;28:25.
16. Connell JT, Sherman WB. Skin sensitizing antibody titer. III. Relationship of the skin sensitizing antibody titer to the intracutaneous skin test, to the tolerance of injections of antigens, and to the effects of prolonged treatment with antigen. *J Allergy* 1964;35:169.
17. Connell JT, Sherman WB. The effects of treatment with the emulsions of ragweed extract on antibody titers. *J Immunol* 1963;91:197.
18. Wide L, Bennich H, Johansson SGO. Diagnosis of allergy by an in vitro test for allergen antibodies. *Lancet* 1967;2:1105.
19. Evans R, Reisman RE, Wypych JI, et al. An immunologic evaluation of ragweed sensitive patients by newer techniques. *J Allergy Clin Immunol* 1972;49:285.
20. Bernstein IL. Experience with RAST in the diagnosis and management of inhalant allergy. In Evans, ed. *Advances in Diagnosis of Allergy: RAST*, Miami, Florida: Symposia Specialists; 17, 1975.
21. Fadal RG and Nalebuff DJ. A study of optimum dose immunotherapy in pharmacological treatment failures. *Arch Otolaryngol* 1980;106:38.
22. Nalebuff DJ, Fadal RG. *In vitro* Determination of initial immunotherapy dosage—a new clinical application of the radioallergosorbent test. In Johnson F, ed. *Allergy: Including IgE in Diagnosis and Treatment*. Miami, Florida: Symposia Specialists; 1979.
23. Nalebuff DJ, Fadal RG, Ali M. Determination of initial dose for ragweed hypersensitivity with Modified radioallergosorbent test. *Otolaryngol Head Neck Surg* 1981;89:271.

24. Young SH. Use of the Modified RAST to determine initial immunotherapy dose. In Fadal, Nalebuff, eds. *RAST in Clinical Allergy* Miami, Florida; Symposia Specialists; 1981:217.
25. Santrach PJ, Parker JL, Jones RT, et al. Diagnostic and therapeutic applications of a modified radioallergosorbent test in comparison with conventional radioallergosorbent test. *J Allergy Clin Immunol* 1981;67:97.
26. Trevino RJ. IgG levels after treatment with antigen based on the scratch testing, intradermal testing, modified RAST testing. *Otolaryngol Head Neck* 1986;95:307–311.

8

Food Allergies and the Role of In Vitro Assays in Their Diagnosis

RICHARD J. TREVINO, M.D.

One of the most enigmatic areas in clinical allergy and immunology is food sensitivity. This chapter will examine the use of *in vitro* techniques in the diagnosis and treatment of food sensitivities.

In 1963, Gell and Coombs[1] classified the various immune mechanisms into four basic types: (1) anaphylaxis, or immunoglobulin E (IgE)-mediated; (2) cytotoxic damage; (3) antigen antibody complexes (both IgG-mediated and IgM-mediated); (4) delayed hypersensitivity (T-cell mediated). All four Gell and Coombs reactions are suspected in the production of the different types of food sensitivities.[2] In fact, it is most likely that all four of the immunologic mechanisms are stimulated simultaneously by food antigens, but the reaction that causes the most severe symptoms is the one that is usually recognized clinically.

Clinically, two types of food allergies occur that involve the immune system.[2] The first is IgE-mediated—Type I anaphylactic reaction, (fixed) food allergy. The adverse reaction occurs within minutes to hours. Symptoms produced are the anaphylactic type and normally occur after ingestion of the food and can include urticaria, hives, angioedema, edema of the face, laryngeal edema, rhinitis, and asthma. These can develop either alone or in any combination. The patients are usually cognizant of this reaction and the cause-and-effect relationship to the offending food. Every time the food is eaten, the symptoms develop and the patient knows which food caused the symptoms. The treatment for IgE-mediated food sensitivity is elimination of the offending food from the diet. Sensitivity to the food usually persists for more than two years after its elimination,[2] though it may last indefinitely. This is especially so with such foods as nuts, fish, and shellfish, which last a lifetime.

The second type of food allergy is the delayed sensitivity, or cyclic food type of allergy, which is non IgE-mediated. Cyclic food allergy has been estimated to account for 80% of the food sensitivity problems seen in clinical practice.[2] These latter sensitivities are more likely to be IgG-mediated and may represent an immune-complex type disease. Unlike fixed food allergies, cyclic food allergies are exposure dependent. The more frequently a food is eaten, the higher the concentration of specific IgG immune complexes. These high concentrations lead to symptoms of food allergy. When exposure is present at nearly every meal, as with such common foods as corn or milk, a small amount of food may actually relieve symptoms for a short period of time. Symptoms produced by this type of food sensitivity occur typically 12 to 24 hours after the ingestion of food. These symptoms are more generalized than IgE-mediated food sensitivities, and their delayed onset makes the cause-and-effect diagnosis more difficult. These symptoms range from headache, muscle ache, tension, and fatigue, to exacerbation of allergic IgE rhinitis and asthma. A clinical history geared to detection of food sensitivity is most useful in diagnosing this type of food sensitivity. Those foods that are eaten frequently would be the foods suspect in causing the symptomatology. *In vivo* tests, such as the oral challenge food test, may supplement the history in the diagnosing of this type of food sensitivity. Nonimmunologic adverse reactions to foods, such as lactose intolerance, celiac disease, favism, should be considered in the differential diagnosis.

If food sensitivity which is immunologically derived is divided into IgE-mediated and IgG-mediated immune complex reactions, it would seem that the diagnosis of food sensitivities would be a simple matter of measuring both specific IgE and specific IgG in the serum. This, however, is not the case.

For the minority of food allergies that are IgE-mediated (immediate type of food sensitivities), the radioallergosorbent test (RAST) and RAST analogs for specific IgE to different foods can be performed. An elevation of specific IgE would lead to a strong suspicion of allergy to that food.[3] However, with this type of food allergy, the history is usually sufficient. The diagnosis is made by the patient, for when a certain food such as shellfish is eaten, symptoms occur within minutes of the ingestion. In these cases, the patient learns to avoid that food, because symptoms are produced every time the food is ingested. In such a case, verification by *in vitro* testing may not be necessary. In some cases, IgE is elevated on RAST testing but no symptoms on ingestion of that particular food. Therefore, the patient is not clinically allergic to this food. These test results may be false-positive. Conversely, certain patients have a normal serum IgE level to a certain food, but ingestion of that food produces immediate symptoms. Because the patient's adverse reactions to that food are obvious, the RAST test would be considered a false-negative one. For children and others from whom a history may be difficult to ascertain, specific IgE RAST testing for foods may be helpful in the diagnosis. IgE-mediated food allergy is more common in younger children than in adults; therefore, *in vitro* testing would more likely be positive in children than in adults.[2] Certain patients may experience anaphylactic-type reactions after eating in a restaurant where multiple foods or ingredients have been prepared in the meals, and it would be impossible for the patient to know which ingredient was the culprit. In these patients, *in vitro* testing would be helpful in differentiating which one caused the symptoms. In general, high RAST scores, class IV or greater, correlate well with significant IgE food allergies (as with anaphylaxis), and any anaphylactic deaths associated with food sensitivities would have very high elevations of IgE.

Another phenomenon that occurs in a few patients with IgE-mediated food sensitivities is the delayed occurrence of symptoms 10 to 12 hours after the initial symptoms. Studies suggest that IgG4 may be involved.[4] IgG4 measurement thus has been postulated to be a good tool for diagnosing delayed food sensitivities in these patients. This type of delayed food sensitivity is a delayed phase of IgE-mediated food sensitivities and must not be confused with the non-IgE-mediated delayed food sensitivities for which measurement of IgG4 is not indicated. Clinically, the diagnosis of IgE food sensitivity is made by history. Measurement of IgG4 to diagnose IgE food sensitivities is not warranted.

Non–IgE-mediated food sensitivities are more difficult to diagnose by patient history. If this second type is proven to be IgE-mediated food sensitivities, the measurement of specific IgE or immune complexes *in vitro* might be a helpful diagnostic tool.[5] The difficulty with this approach is that food antigens are absorbed into the system, and stimulation of IgG production and immune complexes occur as a normal phenomenon.[2] Thus, an elevated IgG or immune complex detectable in the serum of a patient does not necessarily mean that that particular food is causing symptoms.

In addition to the above problem, it is not known at the present time what level of IgG would be significant to produce disease. RAST levels do not directly correlate with symptom production. Normal persons may have high levels of specific IgG, and this particular food would not be causing any symptomatology. A lower level of specific IgG might be the culprit food. There is no way at the present to determine what level of IgG to a particular food in a particular patient would be significant in the symptom production.

Lastly, IgG RASTs for foods have been shown to produce highly variable results, even on the same sample of blood tested in different laboratories.[7] This technical difficulty in defining a cutoff for normals versus abnormals and the reproducibility of the currently available testing methods makes IgG tests for foods unreliable at the present time.

Thus, it is felt that *in vitro* testing for IgE foods may not be necessary in adults as a diagnosis can be made on the clinical history alone, while in children and in certain adults where a good history is not available, it might be necessary. In situations where multiple ingredients have been eaten and an anaphylactic reaction has occurred, *in vitro* testing may be the only method that is available to determine which ingredients caused the symptoms. When there has been a fatal anaphylactic reaction and a food is suspected, IgE from the serum of that individual may be diagnostic in determining if a food was the culprit in that situation.

There are several other *in vitro* test modalities that are still under investigation, namely the basophil histamine release test and the ALCAT test.

The basophile histamine release test is an *in vitro* assay performed on anticoagulated whole blood that contains viable basophils. These basophils are the circulating counterparts of the tissue mast cells and respond to challenges with allergens in a similar manner to mast cells, namely, with release of histamine. The allergen induced histamine release is triggered by the cross-linking of IgE molecules by their specific allergens on the surface of the basophils. The bridging of only a few IgE molecules is sufficient, because the biochemical process that follows amplifies the signal, namely, a measurable histamine release occurs. For this reason, the sensitivity of the basophil histamine release is purported to be slightly greater but less specific than that of the RAST or the RAST analogs for those patients who are allergic but do not process measurable amounts of free IgE. For example, in those patients who have an allergic reaction with ingestion of a certain food and have a normal or low specific IgE by RAST testing, the basophil histamine release test may be positive.

The utility of the ALCAT test, as with any other diagnostic test for food sensitivity, depends on the degree of correlation of its results with results of challenges to test foods. The ALCAT test might be useful in diagnosing adverse food reactions in patients without giving any pathologic mechanism by which the foods are affecting the individual. However, it is still at the present time in investigational phase, and studies need to be performed to corroborate these findings.

Conclusions

The diagnosis of food sensitivity is strongly dependent on history and oral challenge food testing. For IgE food sensitivities, history taking may be sufficient, except in young children. For non-IgE food sensitivity, history plus oral challenge food testing is used for the diagnosis. However, a small number of *in vitro* IgE food screening testing may be useful in predicting the risk of severe or fatal anaphylaxis and to diagnose a fatal anaphylaxis at autopsy. Also, a small number of screening IgG food tests may help in predicting which foods would be suspect, in that high IgG levels would indicate a frequent exposure to that food in these patients and these foods might be the ones chosen for the oral challenge testing.

In vitro techniques can be used as confirmation case-by-case, and the interpretation of the test results needs to be made with careful consideration of the total presentation of the patient. New tests, such as the Basophil Histamine Test or the ALCAT test, may also prove to be useful as clinical tools in the diagnosis of food sensitivities. Further studies need to be performed before *in vitro* testing for foods can be widely accepted as definitive diagnostic tools for food sensitivities.

References

1. Coombs RR, Gell PG. Classification of allergic reactions responsible for clinical hypersensitivity and disease. In *Clinical Aspects of Immunology*, Oxford, England: Blackwell Scientific Publications, 1975;761:761.
2. Trevino RJ. Food allergies and hypersensitivities. *Ear Nose Throat J* 1988; 67:42.
3. Hoffman DR, Haddad ZH. Diagnosis of IgE mediated immediate hypersensitivity reactions to foods by radioimmunoassay. *J Allergy Clin Immunol* 1974; 54:165.
4. El Rafei A, Peters SM, Harris N. Diagnostic value of IgG4 measurements in patients with food allergy. *Ann Allergy* 1989; 62(2):94–99.
5. Leary HL, Halsey JF. An assay to measure antigen-specific immune complexes in food allergy patients. *J Allergy Clin Immunol* 1984; 74:190.
6. Brostoff J. *High Correlation of the ALCAT Test Results with Double Blind Challenge in Food Sensitivities.* Presented at the 45th Annual Congress of the American College of Allergy, Nov. 1988.
7. Trevino AJ, Rapaport S. Problems with in vitro diagnosis of food allergy. *ENT Journal* 1990;69(1).

· 9 ·

The Current Status of Allergy Prediction and Prevention in Infancy Using In Vitro Assays

MATT HAUS, M.D.

Since the early 1960s, reports have suggested that the incidence of allergic disease is on the increase.[1-3] While many of these reports have emanated from the developed countries, changes in the epidemiology and incidence of atopic sensitization have also been observed in the developing communities.[4-7] The realization of this trend has focused much of the current research effort on the establishment of methods designed to prevent or modify the development of the allergic response. In line with this epidemiological shift in allergic sensitization, has been a greater understanding of the immunology of the allergic process. In 1967, Gunnar Johannson and colleagues in Sweden, and the Ishizaka's in the USA, independently discovered serum immunoglobulin E (IgE), the immunoglobulin previously referred to as the Reaginic antibody in the medical literature. Elegant *in vitro* immunoassays designed to measure serum IgE concentrations, and alternate allergic markers, rapidly became available on the commercial market. It is now possible to measure and quantify various biological predictive and diagnostic allergic markers with accuracy and reproducibility. This chapter deals with the clinical application and relevance of these *in vitro* assays, with particular reference to the neonatal period and the first year of life.

84

The Principles of Allergy Prevention

The postponement of allergic disease in infancy appears to be associated with a decrease in the severity of ensuing allergic disease in adults.[8] It has therefore seemed rational to suggest that any methods aimed at preventing or even delaying the onset of infantile allergic symptoms should be encouraged,[9] in spite of the considerable cost in time and effort needed for the effective implementation of any prophylactic regimen. Because of these inherent difficulties, this regimen should, however, be reserved only for the "high-allergic-risk" infant.

The fundamental rationale of the prevention of allergic disease in the high-risk newborn is based on immunogenetic principles. The central concept is one of vigorous and total allergen avoidance to prevent atopic sensitization of the genetically predisposed fetus and infant[10] who experiences a transient, vulnerable period of primary immuno-incompetence during the period from conception through early infancy.[11] This immuno-incompetence is associated with a failure of T-suppressor cell function,[12] which in turn leads to discriminatory effects on various cord blood atopic markers at birth.[13,14]

From animal and human experimentation, it has been shown that sensitivity to allergens is determined by the initial exposure to that allergen in early life, and that the primary exposure to ubiquitous allergens modifies the T-cell response to subsequent exposure.[15] The first year of life is therefore central to any preventive initiatives.

The Principles of Allergy Prediction

The accurate identification or prediction of the "high-allergic-risk" newborn is an integral first step in the prevention program. This needs to occur before, or as soon as possible after, conception to allow the mother to practice adequate antenatal prophylaxis through modification of her own environment. The human fetus is able to produce immunoglobulin E (IgE) from the 11th week of gestation.[16] It has furthermore been shown that the unborn fetus is able to mount an intrauterine allergic response to various allergens, which are presumed to have crossed the materno–fetal placental barrier.[13]

Because atopic disease has been shown to be hereditary[17] the "high-allergic-risk" newborn may be identified by using the following techniques: (1) an adequate family history, which focuses on the presence or absence of atopic disease in the prospective mother, her husband and her existing children (i.e., in the first degree relatives of the newborn); (2) the cord blood total polyclonal IgE test. The threshold limits for this test, as well as the reliability of its predictive function, will be discussed below.

If these measures have not been performed at birth, it is possible to monitor the development of specific IgE antibodies to common ubiquitous allergies during infancy, as possible predictors for subsequent allergic diseases. While not optimal, because of the fact that sensitization will have already occurred, it is nevertheless of use in some situations.

The Pathogenesis of the Allergic Phenotype

The pathogenesis of atopic disease in infancy is subject to multifactorial influences. Both multigenetic, hereditary or intrinsic factors and nongenetic, extrinsic environmental and adjuvant factors interact to determine the clinical expression of atopic disease.[18] The genetic factors responsible for the development of atopic disease are closely associated with T lymphocyte function.[19] Nevertheless, environmental and adjuvant factors, many of which effect the integrity of the epithelial exclusion barriers, are ultimately responsible for the phenotypic expression of allergic disease.[15]

Genetic Factors

The Genetic Regulation of IgE

Murine models have shown that IgE responsiveness to specific protein antigens is genetically controlled both by immune response (Ir) genes in the I region of the major histocompatibility complex (MHC) and by non-MHC linked genes, controlling the magnitude of the IgE response (determining the low and high IgE responder phenotypic expression).[20] Tada[21] first showed that the genetic regulation of the IgE responder phenotype was modified by the T-cell system. It has now been further clarified that interleukin 4 (IL-4), a lymphokine produced by the TH_2 CD_{4+} lymphocyte subset can stimulate the switching on of uncommitted B cells to IgE production.[22,23] A countermeasure to this effect, namely the inhibition of IL-4–stimulated IgE production, has additionally been shown to be a function of IFNγ (gamma-interferon),[24,25] a lymphokine produced by the TH_1 CD_{4+} lymphocyte subset. The net magnitude of the resultant IgE response may therefore be determined by the balance in function between the IL-4 and IFNγ producing T-cell subsets.

In newborns, T cells are immunosuppressed,[27,28] with decreased production of IFNγ.[29–32] This could explain why the period of infancy is so important for allergen avoidance prevention initiatives.

Environmental and Adjuvant Factors

In order to set in motion the cascade of events implicit in the Type I allergic response, specific protein antigen is ultimately required to cross-link the Fab terminal ends of corresponding specific IgE antibodies bound to mast cells, basophils, and eosinophils. This implies that allergen avoidance—whether they be aeroallergens, ingestant allergens or parenterally-administered proteins—is the cornerstone of the preventive program during infancy.[33] In addition, certain adjuvant and other host factors seem central to the pathogenesis of atopic sensitization and to the evasion of immunological tolerance to prevalent antigens. These are summarized in Table 9–1.[15]

In some Third World communities, it has been shown that the epidemiology and immunogenetic mechanisms of atopic sensitization do not follow the generally accepted patterns described in First World situations. While genetic factors seem to be partly responsible for this observation,[34,35] it is suspected that environmental and adjuvant factors in the urban and periurban milieu may be of pivotal importance in influencing the pathogenesis of allergic sensitization in urbanizing communities. Studies in South Africa, where First and Third World conditions coexist, have documented significant differences in sensitization rates during infancy and in the predictive relevance of atopic cord blood markers between different ethnic groups.[4,34,35] It seems probable, therefore, that environmental and adjuvant factors impacting for the first time on urbanizing communities can induce a rapid change in the epidemiology of allergic sensitization in traditionally nonatopic rural populations.

Table 9–1   Host and Environmental Factors Associated with Evasion of Immunological Tolerance to Inhalant Allergens[5,15,33]

RISK FACTOR	POSSIBLE MECHANISM(S)	ADDITIONAL COMMENTS
NO_2[47]	Respiratory epithelial damage[48]	Other air pollutants, including diesel particulates, promote 2° IgE responses[49]
Flu and RSV virus[50]	Respiratory epithelial damage; also effects T-cell function[51,52]	RSV promotes 2° IgE responses[53,54]
Pertussis antigen[55,56]	Affects T-cell function[57]; increases vascular permeability[58]	Pertussis vaccination may effect allergic sensitization
Estradiol[47]	Macrophage function[59,60]; lymphocyte functions[61]; increase TGF production[62]	Dosage as low as 50 μg are effective in adult rats (McMenamin, in press)
Histamine[47]	Increases vascular and epithelial permeability	Mimic effects of "bystander" immune responses
Microbial flora[47]	T-cell function[63]	Effects restricted to certain genetic backgrounds
Immaturity[64]	Immaturity of regulatory T-cell system; immaturity of accessory cells (see discussion)	Oral tolerance also inoperative in newborn mice[46]
Cigarette smoking[65]		
Urbanization[5]		

Prediction of the "High-Allergic Risk" Phenotype

Identifying the High-Risk Newborn

THE ATOPIC FAMILY HISTORY

The high-risk pregnancy may be identified by an adequate family history, which focuses on the presence or absence of atopy in the prospective mother, her husband, and her existing children. Kjellman[36] has laid down clear probability guidelines for the risk of atopic development in offspring who have an atopic family history. These statistics show that the family history of the unborn infant is a good predictor of allergy in its future lifetime, and that the risk of allergic disease for the unborn baby increases with increasing numbers of close relatives with allergy. Table 9–2 denotes the principles of the family score assessment, recommends which newborns need the cord blood *in vitro* test at birth, and clarifies which newborns need to embark on the preventive program during infancy.

NEONATAL PREDICTIVE IN VITRO TESTS

With regard to the identification of the "high-allergic-risk" newborn, the concentration of total serum IgE in newborns has been used as a predictive atopic marker in newborns.[13,14,37] These studies have suggested that newborns with raised cord blood IgE concentrations are at significant risk of developing future atopy. The neonates are advised to adopt the preventive regimen during infancy. Controversy currently surrounds the exact predictive cutoff threshold level for the cord blood IgE concentration, above which

Table 9–2   Family Score Assessment*

FAMILY SCORE	ALLERGIC RISK TO FETUS AND NEWBORN	NECESSITY FOR IgE CORD BLOOD TEST AT BIRTH	NECESSITY FOR PREVENTIVE PROGRAM
0	Minimal risk	No	No
1–3	Possible risk	Yes	Yes: during pregnancy, and then depending on cord blood IgE concentration
4 and over	Very strong risk	Only of academic interest, and as a baseline reference value	Yes: before conception, during pregnancy and after birth, irrespective of the result of the cord blood IgE concentration

*Scoring is as follows: 2 points-mother, father or a sibling with a medically confirmed allergic disease; 1 point—mother, father or sibling with a medically unconfirmed, but suspected, allergic disease; 0 points—mother, father or sibling with no allergic disease.

level the newborn is "at risk." Values of 0.02 ku/L,[34] 0.5 ku/L[37] and 0.9 ku/L[14] have been proposed. Recently, there have been reports questioning the predictive value of cord blood IgE determination. Merrit et al,[39] Hide et al[40] and Ruiz et al[41] have all found cord blood serum IgE an insensitive predictor for future atopic disease, primarily because of the absence of an accepted and reliable threshold cutoff value. Nevertheless, the reports of Merrit and Hide came to these conclusions using "eczema" and "wheezing" as the atopic endpoints during infancy. Studies in newborns, using a combination of a broad range of well defined clinical spectra, and also objective immunological criteria (RAST positivity during infancy) showed clear differences in the cord blood total IgE concentrations between those infants who became sensitized during infancy, and those who did not.[4,34,35] There was not, however, a reliable threshold cutoff level for the cord blood IgE concentrations to differentiate the high-risk newborns, although these studies were not specifically designed to do so. A cutoff level of 0.2 ku/l seems to be the most acceptable for practical usage until this issue is resolved.

Other potential cord blood atopic markers, such as anti-bovine milk-specific IgG[42,34] total eosinophil counts[43] and platelet counts,[44] have been suggested as additional potential atopic markers. At present the predictive relevance of these atopic markers is being assessed.

Cord Blood IgE Assays

There are many different methods for assaying IgE. One requirement is that the assay should be standardized to the World Health Second International Reference Preparation 75/502 of human serum immunoglobulin E. Any kit not so standardized should not be considered. The detection of IgE in serum from cord blood samples requires an ultrasensitive test.[35] Many of the commercially available assays are not sensitive enough to perform reliably. Some manufacturers have produced special low-range procedures for their assays (to improve the detection limit), as the mean expected serum IgE value in neonates is 0.2ku/L, with a range at 1 Standard Deviation of 0.5ku/L, and at 2 SD of 1.3ku/L.

Cord Blood Specific IgE Assays

The most effective laboratory method to assay for specific IgE concentrations in the cord blood is by using a supersensitive, double overnight incubation modification of the Phadebas/Kabi Immunocap RAST assay.[35]

Assay of Specific IgE Concentrations During Infancy

There are many different laboratory assays and systems available to access IgE specific antibodies. Skin tests remain the cornerstone of *in vivo* estima-

Table 9-3   Allergosorbent Tests Reported in the Diagnostic Allergy Survey of the College of American Pathologists

COMPANY	SYSTEM	ALLERGOSORBENT	ANTI-IgE LABEL	STANDARD	SCORING SYSTEM
Pharmacia	Immuno Cap	Hydrophilic polymer	Enzyme	WHO Total IgE	0 to 6
	Phadabas (PRU)	Paper disk	125_1	Birch	0 to 4
	Modified RAST	Paper disk	Emzyme	Total IgE (25IU)	0 to 6
Kallestad	EAST	Paper disk	Enzyme	Rye grass or total IgE (25IU)	0 to 4 or
(Sanofi)				IgE (25IU)	0 to 6
	Modified RAST	Paper disk	Enzyme or 125_1	Total IgE (25IU)	0 to 6
MAST Immuno Systems	MAST	Cellulose threads	Enzyme (luminescence)	2 external controls	0 to 4
Ventrex (Hycor)	Modified RAST	Paper disk	Enzyme 125_1	Total IgE (25IU)	0 to 6
3M Diagnostics, now Whittaker Diagnostics	FAST	Plastic surface	Enzyme (fluorescence)	Rye grass	0 to 4 or 0 to 6

tions, while the *in vitro* methods are all derivatives of allergosorbent tests (AST). Table 9–3 lists the seven allergosorbent tests currently reported in the Diagnostic Allergy survey of the College of American Pathologists.[45,46] The development of specific IgE antibodies to common ingestant and inhalant antigens (such as egg or house-dust-mite allergen) during infancy, is often the first indication of subsequent allergic disease. In this context, these tests can be useful predictive markers for atopy during infancy.

Specific Preventive Initiatives

With the preceding considerations as the background rationale for the specific preventive measures advocated for the "high-allergic-risk" pregnancy and newborn, the following recommendations currently apply.[68]

Planning the Time of Conception and Birth

Recent evidence has indicated that babies who are born in the spring, when the pollen season is at its peak, have developed a higher incidence of allergic disease than babies born in a season when there is a low environmental count of pollen.[66] It may, therefore, be a worthwhile preventive factor to plan the projected date of conception and the subsequent birth of the infant to avoid the spring pollen season. This may be a particularly important preventive measure in those families who have a family score of 4 or more (Table 9–2).

Modification of the Pregnant Mother's Diet

Much controversy has surrounded the role of the mother's diet while she is pregnant, as to the effect of transplacental passage of allergens on the possible causation of allergy in the newborn. Swedish researchers have recently come up with new evidence to show that a mother's diet while she is pregnant did not influence the pattern of allergic disease in her offspring,[67] but other scientists disagree.

In the past, the main principle during pregnancy was to manipulate the diet of the mother so as to prevent allergic foods from making contact with the high-allergic-risk unborn foetus. The current recommendation is for the pregnant mother to ingest whatever balanced diet she feels is recommended for pregnancy in general, but to exclude highly allergenic foods from her diet if possible.

The other important preventive step the pregnant mother should take is to avoid inhaling cigarette smoke. This also means the avoidance of other people's cigarette smoke (passive smoking). Exposure of the fetus to the effects of cigarette smoke by the pregnant mother causes increased levels of IgE in the cord blood of the newborn, and an increased risk of allergy in infancy and childhood.

Feeding Methods in the Infant

MILK FEEDS

The ideal method of feeding for the high-allergic-risk baby in the first six months after birth is to give him or her the benefit of breast milk only. The emphasis on breast milk alone for six months is eminently possible with a little help from the doctor, the midwives and nurses, the local clinic, or the trained nursing aides. The help of a dietitian may also be needed. They will encourage and support the nursing mother.

If the baby's weight gain is inadequate, a milk supplement such as Nutramigen may be added. Nutramigen is a protein hydrolysate substitute containing protein, carbohydrate and fat in the correct proportions for a growing infant, but it is potentially less allergenic than a cow's milk formula. Cow's milk, in any form, must be strictly avoided in the first six months for the reasons stated above.

Breast feeding should be continued for as long as possible after the initial six months critical period. Should breast feeding not be possible, then a hypoallergenic milk with a low potential for causing allergy should be used until one year of age.

SOLIDS

Ideally, no solids should be introduced during the first six months of life. After six months of age, the stepwise and gradual introduction of relatively nonallergic solid foods is allowed: rice, barley, cereal, pears, veal, turkey, lamb. Allergenic foods such as dairy products, fish, eggs and citrus fruits should be avoided in the first year of life.

The mother should be reminded that a pediatrician's or dietitian's advice and help may be needed in planning a nonallergic diet for the infant. As for all healthy and growing babies, a regular check should be made on weight gain.

DIET AND THE BREAST FEEDING MOTHER

Allergens in foods eaten by the breast-feeding mother can be secreted in her breast milk and thereby find their way to the breast-fed baby. While it has not been conclusively shown that the mother's diet while breast feeding adversely affects the lactating infant in the long term, in some individual cases, it is clear that the mother's diet can directly cause eczema and other forms of food allergy in her infant through the excretion of harmful allergens in her breast milk. It is, therefore, advisable that the breast feeding mother should restrict her diet to exclude highly allergenic foods.

ENVIRONMENTAL MANIPULATION AND CONTROL

Environmental allergens should be rigorously excluded from the baby's environment. Strict exclusion of birds and furry animals such as cats, dogs, and rodent pets from the house is mandatory. If a dog is necessary for security reasons, it should be kept outside at all times. Cockroaches and household pests such as rats and mice should be eradicated. House-dust control measures, with frequent vacuum cleaning of bedding and the bedroom, as well as the judicious use of acaricides, should control mite exposure. House moisture removal or desiccation should minimize mould and mite growth.

NON-SPECIFIC ENHANCING FACTORS FOR ALLERGY

It is important to minimize the effect of nonspecific adjuvant enhancing factors for allergy. Parental smoking should be discouraged as a general principle. The 3-in-1 diphtheria tetanus (DPT) inoculation should possibly be delayed because of its adjuvant effect on IgE stimulation. Respiratory viral infections should be minimized. In this regard, overpopulated day care centers are not recommended for high-allergic-risk infants, nor is indiscriminate kissing of the baby by well-meaning friends to be encouraged.

ALLERGY PREVENTION USING MEDICATION

It has been clearly shown that, by delaying the onset of early allergic conditions, the risk and severity of subsequent allergic disease can be minimized. In this regard, researchers have recently shown that, in high allergic risk infants who already had signs of eczema, the administration of a drug called Ketotifen* helped to prevent the development of subsequent asthma in many instances.[69] Furthermore, in young children with chronic chest symptoms, Ketotifen usage resulted in the need for less additional medication and doctor's consultations.[70]

It seems, therefore, that in high allergic risk infants and children who are already showing signs and symptoms of allergic disease (such as eczema) the use of Ketotifen can significantly delay the progression of the allergic process by preventing more serious allergic conditions, such as asthma.

Conclusion

While many of the concepts addressed in this review are controversial, and occasionally confusing, it is nevertheless true that the development and severity of allergic disease can be modified and influenced. While misconceptions and misguided attitudes regarding the diagnosis and management of the "high allergic risk" newborn still prevail, a better understanding of the complex immunogenetic parameters at play in the development of allergic sensitization has provided the platform for more rational guidelines.

---

*Not available in the U.S.

References

1. Glaser J. The dietary prophylaxis of allergic disease in infancy. *J Asthma Res* 1966;3:199.
2. Massicot JG, Sheldon G, Cohen SG. Epidemiologic and socio-economic aspects of allergic diseases. *J Allergy Clin Immunol* 1986;78:954–58.
3. Denis J, Perdrizet S, Levallois M. Increased frequency of allergic diseases in Parisian students from 1968 to 1982 (abs). In *International Symposium on Prevention of Allergic Disease, Florence*. Firenze, Italy: O.I.C. Medical Press, 1984;93.
4. Haus M, Heese H de V, Weinberg EG, Potter PC, Hall JM, Malherbe D. Genetic and environmental influence on cord blood serum IgE and on atopic sensitisation in infancy. *S Afr Med J* 1990;77:7–13.
5. Haus M. Urgent dietary intervention required in urbanising communities to prevent allergy epidemic (letter). *S Afr Med J* 1992;81:117.
6. Turner KJ, Dowse G, Woolcock A. Prevalence of asthma in village communities of the eastern highlands of Papua, New Guinea (abs). In *International Symposium on Prevention of Allergic Disease, Florence*. Firenze, Italy: O.I.C. Medical Press, 1984; 73.
7. Turner KJ, Dowse GK, Stewart GA, Alpers MP. Studies on bronchial hyper reactivity, allergic responsiveness, and asthma in rural and urban children of the highlands of Papua, New Guinea. *J Allergy Clin Immunol* 1986;77:558.
8. Bjorksten B. Does breast feeding prevent the development of allergy? *Immunol Today* 1983; 4:215–217.
9. Businco L, Cantoni A. Prevention of atopy—correct concepts and personal experience. *Clin Rev Allergy* 1984;2:107–123.
10. Bazaral M, Orgel HA, Hamburger RN. IgE levels in normal infants and mothers and an inheritance hypothesis. *J Immunol* 1971;107:794–801.
11. Matthew DJ, Taylor B, Norman AP, Turner MW, Soothill JR. Prevention of eczema. *Lancet* 1977;1:321–324.
12. Bjorksten B, Juto P. Immunoglobulin E and T-cells in infants. In Ganderton M., Kerr JW, eds. *Proceedings of XI International Congress of Allergology and Clinical Immunology*. London: Macmillan, 1983:139.
13. Michel FB, Bousquet J, Coulamb Y, Robinet-Levy M. Prediction of the high allergic risk newborn. *International Allergy Symposium Proceedings*, Uppsala, Sweden. 1980:35–47.
14. Kjellman N-IM, Croner S. Cord blood IgE determination for allergy prediction: a follow up to seven years of age in 1651 children. *Ann Allergy* 1984;53:167–171.
15. Holt PG, McMenamin C, Nelson D. Primary sensitisation to inhalant allergens during infancy. *Pediatr Allergy Immunol* 1990;1:3–13.
16. Miller DL, Hirvonen T, Gitlin D. Synthesis of IgE by the human conceptus. *J Allergy Clin Immunol* 1973;52:182–188.
17. Cooke RA, van der Veer A. Human sensitisation. *J Immunol* 1916;1:201–237.
18. Soothill JF. Some intrinsic and extrinsic factors predisposing to allergy. *Proc R Soc Med* 1976;69:439–442.
19. Del Prete G. Human Th_1 and Th_2 lymphocytes: their role in the pathophysiology of atopy. *Allergy* 1992;47:450–455.
20. Katz DH. Recent studies on the regulation of IgE antibody synthesis. *Immunology* 1980; 41:1–24.
21. Tada T. Regulation of reaginic antibody formation in animals. *Prog Allergy* 1975;19: 122–194.
22. Savelkoul HF, Termeulen J, Coffman RL et al. Frequency analysis of functional IgE-epsilon gene expression in the presence and absence of IL-4 in murine B cells from high and low IgE responder strains. *Eur J Immunol* 1988;18:1209–1215.
23. Pene J, Rousset F, Briere F et al. IgE production by normal human B Cells induced by alloreactive T-cells clones is mediated by IL-4 and suppressed by IFNγ. *J Immunol* 1988; 12:18–24.
24. Finkelman FD, Katona IM, Mosmann TR et al. IFNγ regulates the isotypes of Ig secreted during *in vivo* hormonal immune responses. *J Immunol* 1988; 140:1022–1027.
25. Lundgren M, Persson V, Larsson P, et al. IL-4 induces synthesis of IgE and IgG4 in human B cells. *Eur J Immunol* 1989;19:1311–1315.
27. Hayward AR, Lawton AR. Induction of plasma cell differentiation of human fetal lymphocytes: evidence for functional immaturity of T and B cells *J Immunol* 1977;119:1213–1217.

28. Durandy A, Fischer A, Griscelll C. Active suppression of B-lymphocyte maturation by two different newborn T-cell subsets. *J Immunol* 1979; 123:2644–2649.
29. Bryson YJ, Winter HS, Gard ST, et al. Deficiency of immune IFNγ production by leucocytes of normal newborns. *Cell Immunol* 1980;55:191–200.
30. Lewis DB, Larson A, Wilson CB. Reduced IFNγ mRNA production in human neonates. *J Exp Med* 1986;163:1018–1023.
31. Wilson CB, Westale J, Johnston L, et al. Decreased production of IFNγ by human neonatal cells. *J Clin Invest* 1986;77:860–867.
32. Wakasugi N, Virelizier JL. Defective IFNγ production in the human neonate, I. Dysregulation rather than intrinsic abnormality. *J Immunol* 1985;134:167–171.
33. Haus M. The prevention of allergic disease. *S Afr J Cont Med Ed* 1987;5:37–47.
34. Haus M. Genetic and environmental influences on cord blood atopic markets and an atopic sensitisation in infancy. MD Thesis. University of Cape Town 1988.
35. Haus Heese H de V, Weinberg EG, Potter PC, Hall JM, Malherbe D. The influence of ethnicity of atopic family history and maternal ascariasis on cord blood serum IgE concentrations. *J Allergy Clin Immunol* 1988;82:179–189.
36. Kjellman N-IM. Prediction and prevention of atopic allergy. *Allergy* 1982;37:463–473.
37. Michel FB, Bousquet J, Creillier P, Robinet-Levy M, Coulomb Y. Comparison of cord blood immunoglobulin E concentrations and maternal allergy for the prediction of atopic diseases in infancy. *J Allergy Clin Immunology* 1980;65:422–430.
38. Chandra RK, Pur S, Cheema PS. Predictive value of cord blood IgE in the development of atopic disease and role of breast feeding in its prevention. *Clin Allergy* 1985;15:517.
39. Merrit T, Burr M. Is the determination of cord blood total IgE levels any value in the prediction of atopic disease? (letter). *Clin Exp Allergy* 1992;22:506.
40. Hide DW, Arshad SH, Twuselton R, Stevens M. Cord blood IgE an insensitive method for the prediction of atopy. *Clin Exp Allergy* 1991;21:739–743.
41. Ruiz RGG, Richards D, Kemeney DM, Price JF. Neonatal IgE: a poor screen for atopic disease. *Clin Exp Allergy* 1992;21:467–472.
42. Dannaeus A, Johansson SGO, Foucard T. Clinical and immunological aspects of food allergy in childhood. II. Development of allergic symptoms and numeral immune response to foods in infants of atopic mothers during the first 24 months of life. *Acta Paediatr Scand* 1978; 67:497–504.
43. Haus M, Hall JM, Heese H de V, Weinberg EG, Berman D. Cord blood and maternal total eosinophil counts in relation to infant allergy. *Pediatr Allergy Immunol* 1992;3:23–27.
44. Haus M, Heese H de V, Weinberg EG, Hall JM. Cord blood eosinophils and platelets as predictive atopic markers. *Clin Exp Allergy (abs)*. 1990;20:10.
45. Diagnostic Allergy Survey Set. 1990. CAP Surveys. College of American Pathologists, 1990.
46. Smith TF. Allergy testing in clinical practice. *Ann Allergy* 1992;68:293–301.
47. Holt PG, Britten D, Sedgwick JD. Suppression of IgE responses by antigen inhalation studies on the role of genetic and environmental factors. *Immunology* 1985;62:586–594.
48. Ranga V, Kleinerman J, Collins AM. The effect of nitrogen dioxide on tracheal uptake and transport of horseradish peroxidase in the guinea pig. *Am Rev Respir Dis* 1980;122:483–490.
49. Takafuji S, Suzuki S, Koizumi K, et al. Diesel exhaust particulates inoculated by the intra nasal route have an adjuvant activity for IgE production in mice. *J Allergy Clin Immunol* 1987; 79:639–645.
50. Holt PG, Vines J, Bilyk N. Effect of influenza virus infection on allergic sensitisation to inhaled antigen. *Int Arch Allergy Appl Immunol* 1988;86:121–123.
51. Frick OL, Brookes DL. Immunoglobulin E antibodies to pollens augmented in dogs by virus vaccines. *Am J Vet Res* 1983;44:440–445.
52. Mims CA. Interactions of viruses with the immune system. *Clin Exp Immunol* 1986;66:1–16.
53. Leibovitz E, Freihorst J, Pledra PA, Ogra PL. Modulation of systemic and mucosal immune responses to inhaled ragweed antigen in experimentally induced RSV infection. *Int Arch Allergy Appl Immunol* 1988;85:112–116.
54. Welliver RC, Wong DT, Sun M, Middleton E, Vaughn RS, Ogra PL. The development of respiratory syncytial virus-specific IgE and the release of histamine and nasopharyngeal secretions after infection. *N Engl J Med* 1981;305:841.
55. Haus M, Weinberg EG, Malherbe D. The development of specific IgE antibodies to bordetella pertussis following immunisation in infancy (letter). *Lancet* 1988;1:711.
56. Haus M, Weinberg EG. Specific IgE antibodies to bordetella pertussis after immunisation in infancy (letter). *Lancet* 1988;1:1393.

57. Hirashima M, Yodoi J, Ishizaku K. Formation of IgE binding factors by rat T lymphocytes. II. Mechanisms of selective formation of IgE potentiating factors by treatment of Bordetella pertussis vaccine. *J Immunol* 1981;127:1804–10.

58. Linthicum DS, Munoz JJ, Blaskett A. Acute experimental autoimmune encephalomyelitis in mice: adjuvant action of bordetella pertussis is due to vasoactive amine sensitisation and increased vascular permeability of the central nervous system. *Cell Immunol* 1982;73: 299–310.

59. Slijivic VC, Clark DW, Warr GW. Effect of eostrogens and pregnancy on the antibody response in mice. *Clin Exp Immunol* 1975;20:179–184.

60. Mowat A, Parrott DMV. Immunological responses to fed protein antigens in mice. IV. Effects of stimulating the RES on oral tolerance and systemic immunity to ovalbumin. *Immunology* 1983;50:547–554.

61. Kittas C, Henry L. Effect of sex hormones on the response of mice to infection with toxoplasma gondii. *Br J Exp Pathol* 1980;61:590–605.

62. Knabbe C, Lippman ME, Wakefield LM, et al. Evidence that transforming growth factor is a hormonally negative growth factor in human breast cancer cells. *Cell* 1987;48:417–428.

63. Wanremuehler MJ, Kiyono A, Babb JL, et al. LPS converts germ free mice to sensitivity to tolerance induction. *J Immunol* 1982;129:959–964.

64. Holt PG, Vines J, Britten D. Suppression of IgE responses by antigen inhalation: Failure of tolerance mechanisms in newborn rats. *Immunology* 1988;63:591–593.

65. Magnusson CGM. Maternal smoking influences cord serum IgE and IgD levels and increases the risk of subsequent infant allergy. *J Allergy Clin Immunol* 1986;78:898–904.

66. Björksten F, Svoniemi I, Koski V. Neonatal birch-pollen contact and subsequent allergy to birch pollen. *Clin Allergy* 1980;10:585.

67. Fäith-Magnusson K, Kjellman N-IM. Development of atopic disease in babies whose mothers were receiving exclusion diet during pregnancy—a randomised study. *J Allergy Clin Immunol* 1987;80:686.

68. Haus M. Understanding Allergy Prevention. Guidelines for pregnancy and the First Year. Cape Town, South Africa: Mills Litho (Pty) Ltd. 1993.

69. Ikura Y, Naspitz CK, Mikawa H, et al. Prevention of asthma by Ketotifen in infants with atopic dermatitis. *Ann Allergy* 1992;68:233–236.

70. Polverino M, De Sio Y, Santoriello C, et al. A 3 years trial with Ketotifen (KT) in children with chronic respiratory symptoms. *Am Rev Resp Dis* (Suppl) 1992;145:a708.

In Vitro Diagnosis and the Primary Care Physician

HUESTON C. KING, M.D., F.A.C.S., F.A.C.A.

Principles of Testing

The population of the United States today is just under 250 million. The only in-depth survey of the prevalence of allergy in the United States was carried out by the National Institute of Allergy and Infectious Diseases (NISAID) in 1987.[1] The survey identified 17% of the population as actively allergic, and estimated that the actual number was closer to twice that figure, because patients previously treated but no longer under therapy were not included, nor were those under private care by individual practitioners or those whose symptoms were not recognized as allergic. Physicians, especially primary care physicians, will see 50 to 75 million allergic patients. It therefore behooves the primary care physician to perform allergy testing and treatment properly.

The first order of importance is recognition of the allergic patient. Because allergy may be present in 20 to 30% of the population of patients seen in a general family practice, the examining physician should be alerted to the major signs and symptoms of allergic disease. A complete catalog of the possible symptoms indicative of allergy represents an extensive subject in itself. Some allergic stigmata, however, should be apparent to all primary care physicians. Such classic signs as "allergic shiners," Dennie's lines,[2] the supratip crease of the nose and the allergic salute[3] should alert the physician

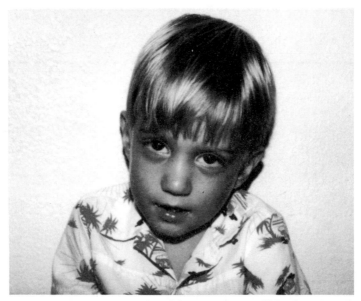

Figure 10–1.   Allergic Shiners. Produced by stagnation of blood in the orbit due to congestion in the nasal mucosa, the dark coloration of the lower lids strongly suggests allergy. (From King HC. *An Otolaryngologist's Guide to Allergy*, New York: Thieme, 1990. Reprinted by permission.)

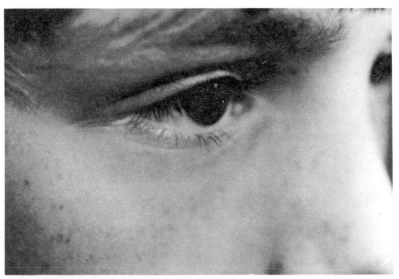

Figure 10–2.   Dennie–Morgan lines. These crescentic lines in the lower eyelid, also known simply as Dennie's lines, result from prolonged spasm in the unstriated muscle of Muller and from poor venous drainage of the orbit due to nasal mucosal congestion, and are typical of allergy. (From King HC. *An Otolaryngologist's Guide to Allergy*, New York: Thieme, 1990. Reprinted by permission.)

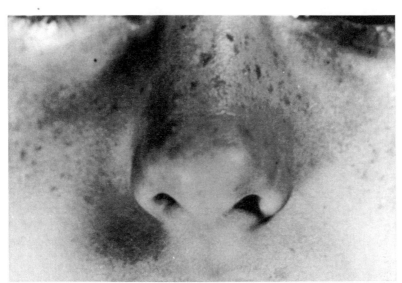

Figure 10–3. Supratip Crease. This skin fold develops after about two years of repeated "allergic salutes" and may become permanent. (Courtesy of Upjohn Co., Kalamazoo, Michigan, Scopes Publications, *Stigmata of Respiratory Allergy*. Reprinted by permission.)

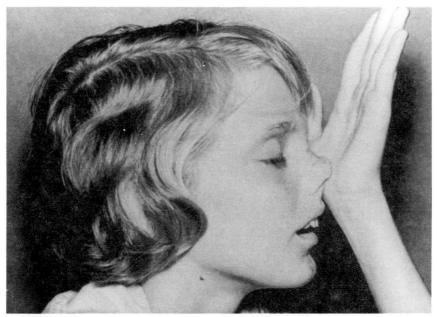

Figure 10–4. The "Allergic Salute." This gesture is commonly seen in the allergic child. It relieves itching and lifts the tip, allowing a breath of air through the congested nose. (Courtesy of Upjohn Co., Kalamazoo, Michigan, Scopes Publications, *Stigmata of Respiratory Allergy*. Reprinted by permission.)

to the probability of significant allergy and institute a course of questioning to expand the picture and confirm the diagnosis.

Approaches to Diagnosis

Allergy, in the broad sense proposed by Clemens Von Pirquet[4] in coining the term, is still diagnosed by history and physical examination. An increasing knowledge of the function of the immune system and the entrance of the laboratory into the realm of diagnosis, however, has made it necessary to further define the diagnostic parameters. Various testing modalities are appropriate only for certain types of allergy, and different forms of therapy may be indicated in accordance with diagnostic findings. Even the term "allergy" has taken on different meanings, and there is not uniform agreement as to the definition of these. In understanding different testing modalities, this lack of uniformity must be understood by the primary care physician if studies are to be evaluated appropriately, and testing and treatment are to be undertaken in an effective manner.

As far as has been determined, most inhalant allergy is mediated by immune globulin E. Since this is the best understood form of allergy, many investigators equate the term "allergy" only with disease produced by immunoglobulin E (IgE), considering all other abnormal reactions as "hypersensitivity." This is not a universally applied definition, however. Most European investigators consider all abnormal reactions involving the immune system in any form as "allergy" and only reactions not involving the immune system as "hypersensitivity." Even here, the definitions are not uniformly applied.[5] Most of the confusion could be avoided if the writer of an article would clarify the definition he is using prior to publication, but this is rarely done. It becomes necessary for the physician attempting to evaluate either the appropriateness of a procedure or the effectiveness of a methodology to try to determine from the context the definitions being used. This may never be truly clear.

As noted, most inhalant allergy is mediated by IgE. This substance is present in the skin, the serum, and the mucus membranes of 20 to 30% of the population in more than trace amounts. This portion of the population is capable of developing inhalant allergy.

Because IgE is present in both skin and serum, either skin testing or immunological analysis of serum IgE is able to measure the amount of IgE present in the patient specific to the allergen in question. There is a degree of difference in sensitivity between skin testing and serum, or *in vitro* testing, but the difference is small. Intradermal skin testing may be the more sensitive of the two, though this may include a larger number false-positive reactions. This increased sensitivity, however, may be offset by the greater specificity for IgE exhibited in *in vitro* testing.[6] Skin testing also allows an inevitable increase in variability of response due to the technique of the person performing the tests. This variability in skin response led to the development of skin endpoint titration (see position statement of the AAOA).[7] Comparable quantification is possible by using *in vitro* testing, and compares well with the pattern seen in skin endpoint titration. Both offer the same format of safety combined with efficiency in starting therapy at as high a dose as is safely possible. The primary care physician can identify the allergens to which his patient is sensitive and determine the degree of sensitivity with very little investment in space or time.

Identifying allergy as the apparent cause of the problem by history and physical examination is, of course, the first necessity. Thereafter, various courses are open. One may wish simply to refer the patient for care to a colleague with an extensive allergy practice. This tends to reduce one's credibility, however, as regional allergy is recognized by the American Board of Otolaryngology as an integral part of the practice of otolaryngology. One may opt for skin testing, but in so doing must be prepared to commit a substantial amount of space and equipment to this part of the practice, as well as developing a greater degree of expertise and technique than is usual in general family practice. Or one may elect to test for individual allergens by *in vitro* methods.

The primary care physician entering the field of *in vitro* allergy analysis today has fewer options than were present a short time ago. In the past, physicians starting an allergy practice could send serum to a licensed reference laboratory with a list of the allergens to be tested, or could provide in-office testing using their own equipment.[8] With the advent of CLIA '88 regulations,[9] the use of in-office *in vitro* allergy testing has become much more complicated. The requirements for in-office laboratory testing are the same as those for a large commercial laboratory. There must be a laboratory director charged with overseeing the activities of the laboratory; however, the clinician may meet the requirements as a laboratory director with proper training and experience. Various professional organizations are in the process of setting guidelines for training in this area. The CLIA requirements are new, and may be expected to undergo extensive revision as time passes.

Fortunately, technological advances have made the CLIA requirements less than prohibitive. While the practitioner might prefer to have the necessary testing equipment in his office, the rapid turnaround provided by most commercial laboratories allows the test results to be available to the clinician nearly as soon as those produced in the in-office laboratory. The cost of obtaining these results has also come down to a level comparable to those practical in skin endpoint titration testing or prick–intradermal testing. In the majority of cases, at the present time, the use of a commercial reference laboratory may be a practical approach to allergy diagnosis by the primary care physician. The primary care physician should be aware of what type of assay for measuring specific IgE the laboratory is using.[10] If the RAST assay is used, the practitioner should know which form of RAST is being used. There are two forms of RAST in common use. The earlier form is the Phadebas

RAST (phRAST). This test concentrated on high specificity to the exclusion of sensitivity, and resulted in having the general allergy community appraising RAST in a negative fashion. Not until the Fadal-Nalebuff Modified RAST (mRAST), which improved sensitivity without significant loss in specificity, did the technique become practical for use in allergy diagnosis and treatment. The mRAST utilizes a 5 class (sometimes a 6 class) format that closely parallels the skin endpoint titration format. This is the format that the clinician must order for proper treatment, and it must be so specified to the laboratory (for correlation to prick-intradermal methods see Chapter 4).

The availability of generally well standardized laboratory results does not relieve the clinician from his duties as a physician. Allergens for *in vitro* testing today number in the hundreds, and no single patient may be expected to be exposed to more than a small percentage of these with any frequency. After the advent of available *in vitro* testing, a brief period ensued in which certain commercial laboratories promoted the use of uncontrolled *in vitro* testing by inexperienced physicians, encouraging the packaged sending of sera with a minimum check list, history, and physical examination. A treatment package would be provided with instructions for use. This resulted in gross overuse of *in vitro* tests, often including hundreds of allergens on a single patient, and the coining of the term "venipuncture allergist." The *in vitro* approach to allergy testing lost much credibility because of this abuse, and even today certain third-party payers are reluctant to provide coverage for *in vitro* testing because of this early overusage of the technique. Such a blanket approach was practiced in skin testing several decades ago, and was discarded. A similar action was necessary in the field of *in vitro* testing.

The largest concern of third-party payers in covering *in vitro* testing was that it cost more than skin testing. The apparent discrepancy was actually based on single skin tests, as in scratch or prick testing, as opposed to quantitative testing by skin endpoint titration. At current costs, there is little difference between commercially provided *in vitro* test results and those identified by skin endpoint titration or skin prick tests. A significant reduction in cost may be provided, however, by taking advantage of screening tests prior to instituting an extensive attempt to identify each allergen affecting a patient. Several years ago, William King[11] established the reliability of a screening battery of tests, employing only the major allergens of the area to both identify the presence of inhalant allergy and direct further study toward the pertinent offenders. While not perfect, the reliability of such an approach is in the high 90th percentile, and provides a cost effective means of proceeding with *in vitro* testing. Most third-party payers have accepted the validity of a screening *in vitro* panel as a precursor to more definitive testing, and, when provided with the information as to the cost effectiveness of the approach, have agreed to recompense the patient for such testing. After determining by screen testing, first, that the patient is in fact allergic to local inhalant offenders, and, second, the specific type of offenders (dust, mold, pollens, epidermals) as indicated by the screen, the testing may be expanded to cover the areas indicated (in conjunction with information provided by the history) to include all of the major allergens necessary to provide adequate relief. In fact, the recommended approach at the present time is to perform a screen of six to ten allergens. Testing for additional inhalant offenders as determined by history is ordered only after a positive screen is obtained. Total IgE is not recommended as a screen but may be used as an adjunct.

There is an alternative approach to screening *in vitro* testing. This involves the use of a technology known loosely as the "dipstick" test. This type of test was designed primarily for use by primary care physicians who do not plan to engage in definitive testing and treatment, but wished to obtain a reliable yes/no answer relative to specific allergens. It is a variation of the ELISA test, and is semiquantitative. Its primary advantage is low cost, a reliable diagnosis of the presence of allergy and to a large extent the allergens involved. The disadvantage is that the test is a qualitative test and therefore treatment cannot be instituted from the results of the test alone. Kits for performing the test are now available from several sources, and it may prove a reasonable means of investigating the relationship of allergy to an individual practice.

A Step-By-Step Approach

The primary care physician considering adding allergy to the practice may well be advised to approach the field through the *in vitro* route. If the primary care physician is unconvinced of the extent to which allergy affects the practice, investing in a limited number of regionally oriented "dipstick" kits may provide the necessary evidence. Once convinced, one may expand practice in the most effective manner by obtaining lists of major regional allergens from one of the allergy supply companies or by following available pollen and mold counts for the area. One may then either select a regional screen for testing, if available, or construct a screen composed of 5 to 15 index allergens prevalent in his area of practice. Even the screen should be dictated by the patient's symptoms, and the seasonal prevalence of allergens conforming to the patient's symptom pattern. A patient complaining of symptoms only in the fall should not be initially tested for trees, which pollinate in the spring. Serum may be sent to a recognized reference laboratory, specifying the allergens to be tested. If all are negative, the problem is most unlikely to be allergy (less than a 1% chance) and pharmacotherapy or other differential diagnoses should be considered. If the tests are positive, a pattern will often emerge indicating not an excessive number of additional tests but an expansion in a particular direction; i.e. seasonal pollens, molds, etc. If needed, a further expansion in allergens tested may be necessary, but progressing toward this in a controlled fashion will do much to control costs without sacrificing needed information.

Once the offending allergens have been identified, treatment must be considered. Unless immunotherapy is contemplated, specific testing is wasteful. If immunotherapy is planned, the primary care physician must be prepared to perform some skin testing to confirm *in vitro* results. It is possible to send laboratory findings to the reference laboratory providing the test results, and request a treatment vial be made. The treatment vial will normally have been made from the same antigens used in performing the *in vitro* tests, and hence should be comparable. Vial testing will still be needed, however. This is covered in Chapter 8; treatment will then be instituted as described in this chapter.

Summary

Based entirely on a consideration of supply and demand, more primary care physicians will be treating allergy patients. A variety of methods are available to make their work clinically competent. It behooves such physicians to be sure that they take full advantage of the available material to keep their work of top quality.

References

1. *Asthma and the Other Allergic Diseases.* NIAID Task Force Report. U. S. Report of Health Education and Welfare. National Institutes of Health Publication No. 79–387, 1979.
2. King HC. *An Otolaryngologist's Guide to Allergy.* New York: Thieme, 1990.
3. *Stigmata of Respiratory Allergy.* Kalamazoo, MI: Scopes Publications, Upjohn Co, 1967.
4. Von Pirquet C. Allergie. *Munch Med Wochenschr* 1906;53:1457.
5. Bahna S. The dilemma of pathogenesis and diagnosis of food allergy, *Immunol Allergy Clin N Amer* 1987:2.
6. Fadal RG, Nalebuff DJ, eds. *RAST in Clinical Allergy.* Miami: Symposia Foundation, 1989.
7. Position Statement, American Academy of Otolaryngic Allergy. Silver Spring, MD, 1987.
8. King HC. *Allergy and the Primary Care Physician,* pp. 36–38. Physician's Marketplace, April 1988.
9. Public Health Service Act (42 U.S.C. 2630) as revised by the Clinical Laboratory Improvement Amendment (CLIA) of 1988, Public Law 100–578.
10. King HC. Allergy testing by primary care physicians. *Postgraduate Med* 1990;87:137–143.
11. King WP. Efficacy of a screening allergosorbent test. *Arch Otolaryngol* 1982;108:81.

· 11 ·

Chronic Sinusitis and
In Vitro Assays

JACQUELYNNE P. COREY, M.D., F.A.C.S., F.A.A.O.A.

Definition of Chronic Sinusitis

Chronic sinusitis can be associated with immune dysfunction by several different mechanisms. Recurrent acute sinusitis may also present a similar picture. For purposes of this discussion, chronic sinusitis will be defined as possessing at least one of the following from each category: (A) nasal obstruction, purulent nasal discharge, chronic cough or headache; and (B) radiologic confirmation of sinus thickening or fluid by plain film, MRI, or CT scan, endoscopic visualization of purulent discharge from the middle meatus or frontal sinus recess, or microbiologic culture positivity from endoscopic, surgical, or antral punctures.

Other diseases that can mimic sinusitis that occur without immunologic dysfunction can include nasal polyposis, cystic fibrosis, midline granuloma, tumors, trauma, congenital cysts (including odontogenic), foreign bodies, and mechanical obstruction of the ostiomeatal complex (Table 11–1).

The question of when to consider immunologic dysfunction clinically may often be a difficult one. Patients who fail standard medical or surgical management, patients with systemic complaints, patients with a history of immune dysfunction, patients at risk for HIV exposure, and patients with signs or symptoms of any of the following clinical syndromes discussed in this chapter should be considered for an immunologic evaluation. The

Table 11–1   Sinusitis and Nonimmunologic
Mechanisms Mimicking Immune Dysfunction

Nasal polyposis
Cystic fibrosis
Midline granulona
Tumor
Trauma
Congenital cysts, including odentogenic
Foreign bodies
Mechanical obstruction of the ostiomeatal complex

thorniest question may be perhaps to determine when "standard" medical therapy for chronic sinusitis has failed. While there is good evidence in the literature to suggest that chronic (greater than two weeks, and up to even six months) administration of antibiotics for otitis media is effective, there is little evidence to suggest that this is beneficial for sinusitis. Despite this, many clinicians empirically give months of antibiotics for recurrent and chronic sinusitis.

Sinusitis and Allergy: (Type I) Immediate Hypersensitivity

The most common association for sinusitis is with immediate type I hypersensitivity, or allergic rhinitis, with or without asthma. The incidence of atopy in the general US population is about 30%. Sinusitis is also among the most common diseases. Sinusitis and atopy are commonly associated, however, whether or not one "causes" the other is controversial. Pelikan and Pelikan-Filipek[1-4] have postulated that mucosal edema and swelling caused by an allergic (type I immediate hypersensitivity) diathesis could cause ostiomeatal complex obstruction, rhinorrhea, and decreased paranasal sinus ciliary action that could then result in the accumulation of mucous and gas in the sinus, with subsequent thickening of the mucosal membrane in the sinuses, a decrease in aeration, increased opacification, and increased air fluid levels and soft tissue mass. They studied 37 patients with nasal provocation challenge and demonstrated both early- and late-phase nasal responses that produced radiographic evidence of mucosal edema and/or opacification. Slavin[5-7] has postulated another mechanism whereby foreign particles become trapped in the mucous of the sinuses where an antigen–antibody interaction with mediator release occurs locally in the mucosal membrane. In further support of these theories is the finding that in a series of patients undergoing surgery for chronic sinusitis, prospective screening with *in vitro* allergy screens for specific-immunoglobulin E (IgE) to routine inhalant allergens and fungi showed a 51 to 57% incidence of positive screens.[8] Numerous other clinical and epidemiologic studies support these theories.[9–19]

Nasal polyps are found more frequently in patients with negative skin tests than in those with positive skin tests. Nasal polyps have an unknown pathophysiology, which may or may not be related to the IgE-mediated mechanism. Settipane[17] also feels that atopic polyp patients have a poorer prognosis by needing more surgical procedures to eradicate polypoid disease. Recent studies by Davis' group also suggest a similar trend.[20] Whether or not allergy "causes" chronic sinusitis, or chronic hyperplastic sinusitis polyps, it is clear that they are often associated. Several techniques exist to identify atopic disease and IgE-mediated immediate hypersensitivity. The oldest and most well-known is of course skin testing. Various methods are available, such as scratch, prick, intradermal, and serial (intradermal) titration testing techniques. These are all quick to administer and easy to read, but require trained personnel and an adequate testing volume to maintain potency of the testing extracts. *In vitro* allergy tests however, can be very useful as screens for these patients. A suggested screening battery might consist of allergens common to the area, such as major weeds, trees, and grass; cats, milk, dust mites, and molds. Total IgE levels are not useful when used alone but when used in conjunction with an *in vitro* screen may be helpful. Elevated total IgE is also helpful to alert the clinician to the possible presence of an "allergic" fungal sinusitis. Routine allergy to fungal antigens also seems to be very common among patients with chronic sinusitis whether or not the syndrome of "allergic" fungal sinusitis is present. Antigens commonly seen include *Candida*, *Aspergillus*, *Alternaria*, *Hormodendrum*, *Cladosporium*, *Helminthosporium*, *Penicillium*, and *Mucor*.

"Mini" and "micro" screens consisting of tests that have, on the same testing disc, a mixture of allergens common to the area are also available for use as screens. A suggested workup for patients with chronic sinusitis is listed in Table 11–2.

The advantage of using a "custom"-designed or specific screen in which all the allergens are known is that if positive, specific advice regarding environmental control for the affected allergens can be provided with specific results. The advantage of micro screens is of course the lowered cost.

Sinusitis and Other Immune Dysfunctions

Sinusitis has also been associated with immunodeficiency states, including AIDS, with systemic immune disorders, and with fungal sinusitis.

Immunodeficiency States

A history of recurrent sinusitis, otitis, bronchitis, meningitis, and/or pneumonia, resistance to routine medical management may suggest a workup for

Table 11-2   Suggested Screening Battery

1. Total IgE
2. a. *Allergen-specific IgE*
        grass
        tree
        weed
        cat
        d. farinae
        d. pteronynissinus
        milk
        molds—*Alternaria, Aspergillus, Cladosporium, Candida*

   Additional molds
        curvularia
        hormodendrum
        tricophyton
        mucor
        penicillium
        botrytis
        stemphyllium
   OR
   b. *Micro screen discs* for regional inhalants

immunodeficiency disorders. Theoretically immune deficiencies can cause infections anywhere, but clinically what occurs are repeated respiratory tract infections. There are several types of immunodeficiencies that have been identified. In Bruton's x-linked agammaglobulinemia, patients do not make antibodies because they lack virgin B lymphocytes. In the hyper-IgM syndrome, deficits in a cell surface protein (CD40) and the T-cell CD40 ligand interaction cause the B-cells to not differentiate properly.

Other syndromes that have been recognized include combined immunodeficiencies (both B and T cells are abnormal), common variable immunodeficiencies, selective IgA deficiency, IgG subclass deficiency and antibody deficiency. The latter is often referred to as "vaccine non-responder state." Again, clinically each of these syndromes present as recurrent upper respiratory tract infections. Unlike patients with severe immunodeficiencies, in whom infections are more fulminant, most of the patients with milder immunodeficiencies have "routine" type infections, but with increased frequency. These subtleties often may be appreciated only after repeated observations taken over a period of time. Another useful clue is repeated surgical failures.

The laboratory evaluation of a patient with suspected immunodeficiency should include both *in vitro* laboratory tests as well as functional antigen stimulation tests. Quantitative, rather than qualitative immunoglobulins should be ordered for the laboratory evaluation of a suspected immunodeficiency. Quantitative levels of IgG, IgA, IgM, IgE and IgD are available by various methods. IgG subclass levels are also available, but one must request the "normal" range reported for each laboratory to properly interpret the result.

A suggested workup, after the method of Richmond[24] is shown in Table 11–3. Quantitative immunoglobulin levels (QIG) for IgG, IgA, and IgM are ordered. IgG subclasses are ordered if the quantitative levels (QIG) are normal. If IgG subclasses are abnormal, order total IgE, IgG subclasses, and a humoral immunity panel. If IgG subclasses are normal and immunodeficiency is still suspected, order the humoral immunity panel. The humoral immunity panel consists of antitetanus antibody (Ab), antidiphtheria Ab, antipneumococal Ab (serotypes, 3, 8, 12, and 14) and antihemophilus influenza B ab. If the humoral immunity panel is normal, no further workup is necessary. If it is abnormal, then immunization with the appropriate antigens (pneumococcus, tetanus, diphtheria) is undertaken. If a repeat humoral immunity panel is normal after immunization, no further testing is necessary. If abnormal, the following tests are suggested: isohemagglutinin titre,

Table 11–3   Laboratory Evaluation of a Patient with Suspected Humoral Immunodeficiency (Id)*

1.0. Quantitative immunoglobulins (QIG) IgG, A, M), (go to 2.0)
2.0.
    2–1. If QIG NORMAL, order IgG subclasses, (go to 3.0)
    2–2. If QIG ABNORMAL, order IgG subclasses and humoral immunity panel, (go to 4.0)
3.0.
    3–1. If IgG subclasses NORMAL and Id still suspected order humoral immunity panel, (go to 4.0)
4.0.
    4–1. If humoral immunity panel NORMAL—STOP
    4–2. If humoral immunity panel ABNORMAL, immunize with appropriate antigens, (go to 5.0)
5.0.
    5–1. Repeat humoral immunity panel—if NORMAL response—STOP
    5–2. Repeat humoral immunity panel—if ABNORMAL—Id, (go to 6.0)
6.0. Obtain: Isohemagglutinin titre
             Anergy profile
             Lymphocyte phenotyping
             Mitogen stimulation (PHA, conA)
             C3, CH50
             Anti-IgA antibody titre
             Pokeweed mitogen

Humoral Immunity Panel
    Antitetanus antibody
    Antidiphtheria antibody
    Antipneumococcal antibody (serotypes 3, 8, 12, and 14)
    Antihemophilus influenzae B antibody

*Sinusitis, otitis, bronchitis, pneumonia, meningitis.

anergy profile, lymphocyte phenotyping, mitogen stimulation with PHA, Con A, pokeweed mitogen, C3, CH_{50} and anti-IgA antibody titres.

Fungal Sinusitis

Chronic sinusitis is also becoming more frequently associated with fungal diseases. Fungal elements can cause several different types of disease, the type and prognosis of which is associated with the immune status of the host. The most common association of fungal disease and chronic sinusitis is the coexistence of chronic infection and atopy to fungal antigens. This is associated, as noted in our previous discussion, by typical signs of perennial allergic rhinitis and atopy to fungal antigens as measured by skin or *in vitro* tests for allergen-specific IgE. Fungal "balls" or fungal colonization may also be present in otherwise normal hosts. Tests of immune function are normal in these patients. "Allergic" fungal sinusitis (AFS) has been reported for *Aspergillus*, *Alternaria*, *Curvularia*, *Bipolaris* species, and *Exserohilium*. *In vitro* tests in these patients show positive allergen-specific IgE to the suspected fungus, a markedly elevated total IgE, and precipitating antibodies (IgG) to the fungal antigens. Skin tests show immediate positive cutaneous reactivity, and sometimes delayed reactivity as well. Histopathologic analysis shows "allergic mucin" with prominent eosinophilia. Charcot–Leyden crystals, and fungal hyphae. Surgical cultures often show a mixed bacterial flora as well. The clinical picture of these patients is that of hyperplastic polypoid sinusitis, usually recurrent, and responsive only to surgery, debridement, and steroids. The main immunologic feature that distinguishes these patients from atopic patients with chronic sinusitis is, however, the presence of precipitating antibodies in cases of AFS.[25,26] Chakrabarti[27] has suggested that these are both part of the spectrum of the same disease and that the presence of precipitating antibodies is a clue to a poorer prognosis. Tests for precipitating antibodies are available from a few laboratories and only for a few fungal antigens (usually *Aspergillus* species). Immunologic diagnosis may be difficult to obtain for many suspected fungal pathogens. Commercially available fungal allergen-specific IgE and total IgE by RAST, ELISA, and other methods are readily available for the most commonly suspected species, *Aspergillus*, *Alternaria*, and *Curvularia*. Invasive fungal sinusitis usually occurs in immunocompromised hosts. It appears to "overwhelm" the immune system so that routine tests, such as total IgE, are normal or often not done due to the patients' grave condition. It may, however, occur in patients with normal immune function as well, but is usually not as fulminant.[25,26] Table 11–4 lists a suggested *in vitro* workup for suspected fungal diseases of the sinuses.

AIDS–Related Immunodeficiency

One last type of chronic sinusitis that may be associated with IgE-mediated disease is the recently reported phenomenon of an allergic rhinitis-like

Table 11–4   Suggested *In vitro* Workup
for Fungal Diseases of the Sinuses

- Total IgE
- Allergen-specific IgE
  To inhalants (grass, trees, weeds, dust mites, cat)
  To specific fungal antigent
    Aspergillus
    Alternaria
    Curvularia
- Allergen specific IgG
    Aspergillus
    Other fungal antigens if suspected
- Precipitating antibodies

syndrome and hyper-IgE syndrome in HIV positive patients. Certain patients with AIDS show a progressive elevation of IgE levels and an associated increase in histamine release.[28]

There appears to be a high incidence of allergic disorders in patients with HIV infection. This is felt by Rubin and Honigberg to help explain the additional association of AIDS and chronic sinusitis.[29] IgG subclass deficiencies may also be noted in AIDS patients. These are clinically associated with not only recurrent sinusitis, but otitis, bronchitis, and pneumonia.[30]

In summary, chronic sinusitis can be associated with immediate type I hypersensitivity. *In vitro* screens for inhalant allergens and fungal allergens/antigens can be useful to identify the presence of atopy to inhalant and fungal antigens in these patients. Chronic sinusitis is also associated with non-IgE mediated immunologic dysfunction, including fungal diseases and immunodeficiency states. A combination of *in vitro* tests of immune function and functional immunologic testing as outlined can be useful to help diagnose these patients. Lastly, chronic sinusitis can be associated with both hyper-IgE disease and IgG subclass deficiencies as well as the more commonly identified lymphocyte subset (CD4) deficiencies in HIV positive patients. *In vitro* determinations of total and allergen specific IgE in these patients can be useful as well.

References

1. Pelikan Z, Pelikan-Filipek M. Role of nasal allergy in chronic maxillary sinusitis: Diagnostic value of nasal challenge with allergen. *J Allergy Clin Immunol* 1990; 86:484–491.
2. Pelikan Z. Chronic sinusitis maxillaris and a possible role of the allergic reaction in the nasal mucosa. *Ned Tijdschr Geneeskd* 1988; 132:329–331.
3. Pelikan Z. Nasal challenge with allergen (NPT) in patients with chronic sinusitis maxillaris. Abstract. *N Engl Reg Allergy Proc* 1988; 9:253.
4. Pelikan Z. Role of nasal allergy in chronic sinusitis maxillaris (CSM): Diagnostic value of nasal challenge with allergen (NPT). Abstract. *J Allergy Clin Immunol* 1989; 83:214.

5. Slavin RG, Zilliox AP, Samuels LD. Allergic sinusitis: Does it exist? Abstract. *N Engl Reg Allergy Proc* 1988; 9:253.

6. Slavin RG. Clinical disorders of the nose and their relationship to allergy. *Ann Allergy* 1982; 49:123–126.

7. Slavin RG. Sinusitis in adults (Symposium). *J Allergy Clin Immunol* 1988; 81:1028–1032.

8. Corey JP, Bumsted RM, Panje WR, Shaw GY, Conley D. Allergy and fungal screens in chronic sinusitis. *Amer J Rhin* 1990; 4:25–28.

9. Jeney GR, Meredith S, Baramiuk J, Kaliner M. Nasal secretions in recurrent sinusitis and otitis. Abstract. *J Allergy Clin Immunol* 1989; 83:214.

10. Lober P. Histology and pathology of the nose and sinuses. In Parparella MM, Shumrick DA, eds. *Otolaryngology* 1983; Philadelphia: WB Saunders, 1:551–62.

11. Middelton E, Jr. Chronic rhinitis in adults (Symposium). *J Allergy Clin Immunol* 1988; 81:971–975.

12. Pearlman DS. Chronic rhinitis in children. *J Allergy Clin Immunol* 1988; 81:962–966.

13. Rachelefsky GS, Goldberg M, Katz RM, et al. Sinus disease in children with respiratory allergy. *J Allergy Clin Immunol* 1978; 66:310–314.

14. Rachelefsky GS, Katz RM, Siegel SC. Chronic sinusitis in children with respiratory allergy: The role of antimicrobials. *J Allergy Clin Immunol* 1982; 69:382–387.

15. Rohr AS, Spector SL. Paranasal sinus anatomy and pathophysiology. *Clin Rev Allergy* 1984; 2:387–395.

16. Sacha RF, Trembray NF, Jacobs RL. Chronic cough, sinusitis, and hyperreactive airways in children: An overlooked association. *Ann Allergy* 1985; 54:195–198.

17. Settipane GA, Chafee FH. Nasal polyps in asthma and rhinitis: A review of 6037 patients. *J Allergy Clin Immunol* 1977; 59:17–21.

18. Shapiro GG, Furukawa CT, Pierson WE, Gilbertson E, Bierman CW. Blinded comparison of maxillary sinus radiography and ultrasound for diagnosis of sinusitis. *J Allergy Clin Immunol* 1986; 77:59–64.

19. Williams HL. Nasal physiology. In Paparella MM, Shumrick, eds. *Otolaryngology*. Philadelphia: WB Saunders, 1983; 1:329–346.

20. Nishioka GJ, Cook PR, Davis WE, McKinsey JP. Immunotherapy in patients undergoing functional endoscopic sinus surgery. *Otolaryngol Head Neck Surg* 1994; 110:406–412.

21. Hanson LA, Soderstrom R, Avanzini A, et al. Immunoglobulin subclass deficiency. *Pediatr Infect Dis J* 1988; 7:17–21.

22. Lai V. *Allergic Rhinitis in Hypogammaglobulinemia*. Presented at the Fall AAOA Meeting; September, 1992; Washington DC.

23. Steiner D, Feehs K, Georgitis JW. Immunodeficiency in children with recurrent sinusitis and otitis. Abstract. *J Allergy Clin Immunol* 1989; 83:276.

24. Richmond GW. *IgG Subclass Deficiency and Chronic sinusitis*. Presented at the Spring AAOA Meeting; May, 1991; Waikoloa, Hawaii.

25. Corey JP, Romberger CF, Shaw GY. Fungal diseases of the sinuses. *Otolaryngol Head Neck Surg* 1990; 103:1012–1015.

26. Corey UP, Seligman I. Otolaryngology problems in the immune compromised patient—An evolving natural history. *Otolaryngol Head Neck Surg* 1991; 104:196–203.

27. Shah A, Khan ZU, Charturvedi S, et al. Allergic bronchopulmonary aspergillosis with coexistent aspergilloma: A long term follow-up. *J Asthma* 1989; 26:109–115.

28. Chernoff D, Sample S, Lenahan G, et al. *A high incidence of allergic disorders in patients with HIV infection*. Proceedings of the 5th International Conference on AIDS. June 1989; Montreal.

29. Rubin JS, Honigberg R. Sinusitis in patients with acquired immunodeficiency syndrome. *ENT J* 1990; 69:460–463.

30. Sample S, Lenahan GA, Serwonska MH, et al. Allergic diseases and sinusitis in acquired immunodeficiency syndrome. *J Allergy Clin Immunol* 1989; 83:190.

· 12 ·

Laboratory Diagnosis of Chronic Fatigue Syndrome and Related Diseases

Lewis L. Perelmutter, Ph.D.

Chronic Fatigue Syndrome

Chronic fatigue syndrome (CFS) is an illness characterized by debilitating fatigue and several flulike symptoms, such as pharyngitis, adenopathy, low-grade fever, myalgia, arthralgia, headache, difficulty concentrating, and exercise intolerance. These nonspecific symptoms can make the syndrome difficult to identify. Profound fatigue—the earmark of the disorder—usually comes on suddenly and persists or relapses throughout the course of the illness. But unlike the short-term fatigue and malaise that often accompany an acute infection, by definition, CFS symptoms linger for at least six months and often for years.

Chronic fatigue is a common complaint in primary care practice. No evidence exists to suggest that most patients with chronic fatigue have CFS. Indeed, CFS is probably an uncommon cause of chronic fatigue.

Most investigators studying CFS believe that the syndrome has many possible causes. For example, various infectious agents often trigger the onset of CFS. Preliminary research also shows a variety of immunologic distur-bances in some patients. No single pattern of disturbances appears consis-tently, however, and in general, patients are not clinically immunocompromised; they do not develop opportunistic infections. In fact, the character, epidemiology, and prognosis of CFS is quite distinct from that of major immune deficiency disorders, such as AIDS. Several different latent viruses also appear to be reactivated in some CFS patients, although reactivation has not been shown in all patients; and it is not clear that any of these viruses is causally related to CFS or its symptoms. Many patients with CFS also present with anxiety or depression. In summary, as with most chronic illness, CFS has both physical and psychiatric manifestations.

Epidemiology

Most cases of CFS are sporadic; the patient does not have a close contact who has developed a similar illness. Infrequently, however, close contacts, including family members, become ill with CFS at about the same time. During the past 60 years, several apparent epidemics of this illness affecting various communities or relatively large numbers of co-workers have been reported. Clusters of CFS cases are unusual, however, and it is not generally thought that people with CFS need to be isolated in any way. The clinical and laboratory findings of sporadic versus epidemic cases have yet to be compared.

While the typical patient seeking medical care for CFS is a white woman in her thirties, patients of all ages (including the very young and very old), both sexes, many races, and all socioeconomic groups have been affected. Centers for Disease Control (CDC) and National Institute of Allergy and Infectious Disease (NIAID) sponsored researchers have studies under way to try to estimate the prevalence of this disorder.

Historical Perspective

Although interest in this illness has grown tremendously since the mid-1980s, CFS does not appear to be a new disorder. It closely resembles neurasthenia or neurocirculatory asthenia, diagnoses commonly made in the late 19th and early 20th centuries. As stated earlier, small epidemics of a very similar illness (most often called myalgic encephalomyelitis, or ME) have been described in the medical literature for at least 60 years. Furthermore, case reports describing similar illnesses date back several centuries. These sporadic cases of fatigue syndromes have often been linked to bacterial, viral, or protozoal infections (for example, brucellosis and influenza). But fatigue syndromes also appear outside the setting of an infectious illness. Several recent studies indicate that the rheumatological disorder called fibrositis or fibromyalgia, first described in the 19th century, is very similar to CFS. The average age of the patient with fibrositis is a bit older, however, and soft-tissue pain is a more prominent symptom in this illness.

In the 1980s, several studies indicated that antibody levels to one virus, Epstein-Barr virus (EBV), were somewhat higher in patients with CFS than in healthy individuals. It is important to put this observation in context. EBV infection is extremely common; approximately 90% of American adults have been infected, and they harbor a lifelong infection thereafter. In most people the virus remains dormant. Antibody studies indicate that EBV may be reactivated—that is, self-replicating—more often in patients with CFS than in healthy individuals. But the difference is not striking. Moreover, as mentioned earlier, evidence shows that several other viruses may also be reactivated in CFS. Therefore, investigators believe that there is no proof that EBV causes CFS, at least in most patients.

Clinical Picture

A hallmark of CFS is the sudden onset of the illness, typically with flulike symptoms. In contrast to the usual flulike illness, however, the symptoms of CFS do not fully resolve; they persist chronically, or wax and wane frequently, accompanied by debilitating fatigue and malaise.

In a few cases, CFS seems to follow from a bout of classic acute mononucleosis rather than from a nonspecific flulike illness. In these cases, EBV—the cause of most cases of acute mononucleosis—may play a role in the pathogenesis of CFS. Clearly some CFS symptoms—headache, myalgia, sleep disorder, difficulty concentrating—could be secondary symptoms of a primary affective disorder. However, other symptoms such as pharyngitis, fever, adenopathy, and arthralgias suggest a different underlying process.

Many patients have a history of allergies years before the onset of CFS, and occasionally allergic symptoms worsen after these patients become ill. Allergies are so prevalent in CFS patients that it is important to differentiate those symptoms that are allergy-related and thus amenable to treatment.

The course of CFS varies greatly, with symptoms lasting anywhere from many months to many years. Symptoms typical of CFS are often seen for short periods of time; but these symptoms must persist for at least six months, according to the current CDC definition, to entertain a diagnosis of CFS. Fortunately, CFS is not a progressive disease; usually the symptoms are most severe in the first year of illness. Systematic studies are under way to better define the prognosis.

Evaluation of Patients

The patient with the complaint of chronic fatigue that is interfering with his or her life must be taken seriously.

CFS symptoms overlap with those of many well-recognized illnesses. For example, Lyme borreliosis, mild systemic lupus erythematosus (SLE), and early or mild multiple sclerosis (MS), are among the numerous disorders that resemble CFS. A history of potential tick exposure, the typical Lyme rash (*erythema chronicum migrans*), and antibodies to the Lyme spirochete suggest the diagnosis of Lyme borreliosis. In both SLE and MS, debilitating chronic fatigue can be more prominent than rheumatologic or neurologic symptoms. Psychiatric illnesses that most resemble CFS include major depressive episode, panic disorder, generalized anxiety disorder, and somatization disorder. It remains unresolved whether prior or current depressive episodes should exclude a diagnosis of CFS.

Although infectious agents can trigger the syndrome, the diagnosis of CFS currently is one of exclusion. The patient's medical history, particularly his or her potential epidemiologic exposures, and physical examination will help determine the need for various laboratory tests. A reasonable initial laboratory workup would include a urinalysis, complete blood count and differential count, chemistry panel, thyroid function test (a TSH test may be sufficient), erythrocyte sedimentation rate, antinuclear antibodies, and rheumatoid factor. Significantly abnormal results on any of these tests should prompt consideration of alternative diagnoses. It is prudent for physicians today to also consider the possibility of infection with the human immunodeficiency virus. Subsequent workup should be guided by the clinical picture and may necessitate a chest X-ray, an electrocardiogram, and IgG level, a tuberculin skin test, and serum cortisol determinations, among other tests.

Immunologic Features

Many different immunologic findings have been described in patients with CFS, but no single immunologic disturbance has yet been identified as typical of the syndrome.

Those disturbances observed include depressed natural killer (NK) cell activity, elevated viral antibody titers, and circulating immune complexes. These findings indicate general differences between patient populations and control groups, but none is specific for CFS or abnormal in all CFS patients.

Neuropsychologic Features

As mentioned earlier, many patients with CFS also meet diagnostic criteria for depression or anxiety disorders at presentation. It remains unclear whether a higher than normal frequency of psychiatric disorders in this patient group also exists in the years prior to the onset of CFS. On the other hand, psychiatric evaluations fail to identify any psychiatric disorders in some patients. Because subtle psychiatric problems can be difficult to recognize, consultation with a psychiatrist or psychologist may benefit the evaluation of some patients.

Many people with CFS have neurological symptoms, including paresthesias, dysequilibrium, and visual blurring. A few patients who are otherwise identical to the larger group have had more dramatic acute and transient neurologic events, such as primary seizures, periods of severe visual impairment, and periods of paresis. These few patients show no evidence of any well-recognized neurologic disorder, such as MS. Patients with these more dramatic symptoms warrant a more intensive neurologic workup.

Preliminary research indicates that some patients with CFS demonstrate punctate areas of high signal in the subcortical white matter on magnetic resonance imaging scans of the brain. Studies are under way to determine if these abnormalities are found more frequently in people with CFS than in healthy individuals.

For many patients, the cognitive impairment they experience is one of the most disconcerting symptoms. It is usually characterized as an inability to concentrate, unusual absent-mindedness, and difficulty with word finding. CFS patients do not exhibit gross dementia. Neuropsychological testing is being conducted to better define the presence, nature, and severity of cognitive impairment in patients with CFS.

Because of CFS' diversity and common symptomatology with many other diseases, diagnosis and management present a real challenge. Below is a laboratory approach that attempts to exclude or include CFS.

If the major and minor criteria are consistent with possible CFS, the next step is a laboratory panel to aid in the exclusion of most of the other chronic–fatigue-producing conditions, including anemias, rheumatoid diseases, and thyroid disease. If this panel does not reveal evidence of other conditions or if the other condition is treated and no progress in the resolution of the chronic fatigue is obtained, then thorough evaluation of the immune system, including immune deficiency, immune activation, and allergy, as well as infectious disease and adrenocortical hormones, should be considered.

Exclusionary tests consist of complete blood count with platelets and differential, reticulocyte count, and sedimentation rate. They should also include an extended chemistry profile along with electrolytes, lead blood level, Lyme serology, urinalysis, throat culture, and tuberculosis purified protein derivative (PPD) skin testing. The exclusionary tests should be done to eliminate rheumatological problems by performing rheumatoid arthritis (RA) latex screen, antinuclear antibody (ANA), and C-reactive protein. Thyroid profile should be determined by running T_4, T_4 uptake, free thyroxine, total T_3, and thyroid stimulating hormone (TSH). A thyroid autoimmune panel with various antinuclear and ribonuclear proteins is also included.

The laboratory procedures for inclusion of CFS are *in vitro* allergy testing for inhalants and foods. They should also include an immunodeficiency panel (Table 12–1), infectious panel (Table 12–2), an immune activation panel (Table 12–3), and a neuroendocrine panel (Table 12–4).

Because some of the procedures discussed above are used frequently and

Table 12–1   Immunodeficiency Panel

Immunoglobulins G, A, M
IgG Subclasses (IgG$_1$, IgG$_2$, IgG$_3$, IgG$_4$)
Antitetanus antibody
Antipneumococcal antibody

play an important role in excluding or including CFS, these methodologies
are discussed in greater detail below.

Epstein-Barr Virus

Within the past 20 years several distinct EBV-related cell-associated antigens
have been characterized by immunofluorescence and other serological procedures. These include EB viral capsid antigens (VCA),[1,2] EBV membrane
antigen, EB nuclear antigen (EBNA),[3] EBV-induced early antigen (EA)[4,5]
(subdivided into restricted [R] and diffuse [D] components), and various
soluble antigens. The first four classes can be demonstrated by immunofluorescence, enzyme-linked immunosorbent assay (ELISA) or immune-
adherence hemagglutination techniques and the last by complement fixation
and immunodiffusion.[6,7] There are also several techniques now available that
can measure the presence of neutralizing antibodies to EBV.[8]

   Serological procedures are utilized for the following reasons: (1) to determine susceptibility or immunity to IM or primary infection; (2) to determine
whether a heterophile antibody-negative mononucleosis syndrome in a patient is etiologically related to EBV (because all cases of heterophile-positive
mononucleosis are due to EBV, it is rarely necessary to measure specific EBV
antibodies as a diagnostic procedure in mononucleosis); (3) to determine
whether EBV can be implicated as the etiologic agent in a variety of clinical
syndromes of unclear etiology, such as hepatitis, encephalitis, infectious
polyneuritis, idiopathic thrombocytopenia, hemolytic anemia, etc., which
have occasionally been associated with EBV infection; (4) to determine
susceptibility or immunity to infection in primates used in experimental EBV
inoculation experiments; (5) to determine whether a lymphoblastoid cell line
contains antigenic markers of EBV expression; and (6) as epidemiological
tools in specific populations (in particular, seroepidemiological methods have

Table 12–2   Infectious Disease Panel

EBV (IgG and IgM to NA and VCA)
HHV-6
HIV Antibody
Candida IgG, IgA and IgM Antibodies

Table 12–3   Immune Activation Panel

Complete Blood Count
Flow Cytometry Determination on:
IL-2 Receptors on CD_4 (Helper Cells)
IL-2 Receptors on CD_8 (Suppressor Cells)
Early and Late T-Cell Activation
T-Cell HLA-DR Marker
NK Cell Marker

been used to distinguish patients with EBV-associated tumors from individuals with routine infection).

Cytomegalovirus

Human Cytomegaloviruses (CMVs) are members of the Herpesvirus group and are ubiquitous. The host characteristically becomes latently infected after the primary infection. An active infection resulting from a primary or reactivated latent infection during pregnancy may be transmitted to the fetus or to the infant during birth. The congenitally infected infant is usually viruric for a prolonged period, with the pathologic consequences ranging from no overt illness to severe central nervous system damage. A primary infection in the adult may be asymptomatic; or various syndromes, including CMV mononucleosis, hepatitis, or pneumonitis, may result. In the immunocompromised patient the clinical consequences of a primary or reactivated latent infection are often life threatening. The natural history of CMV infection has been extensively reviewed.[9]

Seronegative recipients transfused with blood from seropositive donors are at the highest risk of acquiring CMV infection with clinical sequelae; the pathologic consequences are most severe in the immunologically immature or compromised host. The screening of donor and recipient sera for antibody to CMV, therefore, has important implications for patient care.

The presence of active CMV infection can only be inferred from serological data and must be confirmed by viral isolation. Preferred sources for the recovery of virus are urine and saliva, although virus may be isolated from various body secretions and tissues. CMV in urine without preservatives

Table 12–4   Neuroendocrine Panel

ACTH
Cortisol
Dehydroxyepiandrosterone (DHEA)
DHEA-Sulfate (Urine)

retains 90% of its infectivity for one week if transported on wet ice and stored at 4°C. The strict species-specific requirement for *in vitro* replication necessitates the routine use of cultures of diploid human fibroblasts for isolation attempts. Human CMV isolates are identified by the characteristic cytopathic effect (enlarged, round cells with prominent intranuclear inclusions), the species-specific requirements for growth *in vitro*, the absence of significant amounts of cell-free virus during the initial passage in cell cultures, and the application of immunologic procedures. CMV antigens can be detected in infected cells by the indirect fluorescent-antibody (IFA) test by using human immune sera devoid of antibodies to the other herpesviruses. The increasing availability of monoclonal antibodies, however, should supplant the use of human or animal polyclonal antisera. Monoclonal antibodies provide low background and a bright, reproducible fluorescent reaction when used in IFA procedures. They may be used individually, although a mixture of several monoclonal antibodies often provides an improved reaction. Although tedious and time-consuming, the production and characterization of monoclonal antibodies for diagnostic uses is not beyond the capabilities of many laboratories.[10] Monoclonal antibodies to CMV have been used in rapid diagnostic procedures to detect both viral antigen in biopsy specimens[11] and CMV antigen in cell cultures inoculated with clinical specimens and incubated for 36 hr.[12]

A degree of antigenic heterogeneity has been demonstrated between human strains of CMV by using human and animal immune sera. The significance of these findings to diagnostic procedures is not established. Immunologic data based on the use of an antigen prepared from a single strain of CMV may be misleading and should therefore be compared with reference reagents. The demonstration of specific antibody by using commercially available antigens is routine in most diagnostic laboratories.

The complement fixation (CF) test has been commonly used for determining levels of CMV antibody. It is recommended, however, that laboratories initiating CMV serology utilize a more sensitive assay, such as ELISA or the indirect hemagglutination (IHA) test. These tests are available commercially, reliable, and amenable for use in screening large numbers of specimens.

Candidiasis

Latex agglutination (LA), immunodiffusion (ID), and cross immunoelectrophoresis (CIE) tests are valuable in the diagnosis of systemic candidiasis in the immunologically intact host.[13] In contrast, the serodiagnosis of candidiasis by agglutination and CF tests has proven to be of little reliability because of positive responses by healthy subjects or by persons with superficial candidiasis without systemic involvement.[13] Negative results by these tests may be of value in excluding systemic candidiasis as a diagnosis. The quantitative LA and the ID and CIE tests appear to give the most reliable results for antibody detection of systemic candidiasis in immunologically intact hosts. The ID and CIE procedures yield results that are apparently comparable.[13]

Immunosuppressed patients often fail to produce antibodies, so a negative antibody test does not necessarily rule out the disease. Such patients may be in a state of antigen excess, so that tests for antigen will be positive. Encouraging reports from many laboratories indicate that tests, such as enzyme immunoassay (EIA) for *Candida albicans* antigenemia are proving useful for the diagnosis of invasive candidiasis in immunologically compromised hosts.[14] Antigenemia occurs when mannan polysaccharide is sloughed off *Candida* cell walls and persists for a few days in the plasma. Mannanemia has also been observed by researchers using diverse methods of detection in patients with chronic mucocutaneous candidiasis.[14]

Lyme Disease

Several clinically important questions about a patient's possible infection with *Borelia burgdorferi*—the causal agent of Lyme disease—should be answerable by good laboratory tests.

- Has the patient ever been infected with *B. burgdorferi*?
- Is the patient currently infected with this organism?
- How recently did the infection begin?
- Is the patient's current illness related to this infection?
- If a patient has signs and symptoms of autoimmune disease, are they related to an infection with *B. burgdorferi*?
- Has a course of treatment been effective in eradicating infection?

Complexities of the host–organism relationship and insensitivity and nonspecificity of test methods have led to confusion concerning the interpretation and utility of serological tests for Lyme disease.

OVERVIEW OF ANTIBODY RESPONSE TO *B. BURGDORFERI*

The first antibody response to *B. burgdorferi* is of the immunoglobulin M (IgM) class, and it is not usually detectable by the commonly employed ELISA or IFA tests for three to five weeks following infection, if at all. Because the total amount of specific IgM produced is typically minute, many of the routinely performed IFA and ELISA tests for *Borrelia*-specific IgM never turn positive. Published data show only a 30% detection rate by ELISA for IgM antibody in patients with early Lyme disease.[15]

IgM switches to IgG as the humoral immune response proceeds, and if the patient comes to a physician for care some weeks after the initial infection, IgM may no longer be detectable by ELISA or IFA because the absolute amount of IgM has decreased, and the now more plentiful and more tightly binding IgG will compete successfully for and block reagent antigen sites. Therefore, IFA and ELISA tests often cannot distinguish between recent and remote infection.

Very sensitive serological tests may turn temporarily negative because of the formation of immune complexes–a combination of an antibody with its corresponding antigen. For a brief period during a developing antibody response, it may happen that essentially all the specific antibody is bound to circulating antigen and is, therefore, not available to react with test antigen. In this situation, the antibody could be detected only if first dissociated from the complex, such as by the use of reducing agents. Following dissociation, the authors of this recent report demonstrated that some previously negative sera turned antibody-positive.

A major problem with this report, however, was the use of ELISA to judge initial reactivity, followed by a more sensitive Western blot assay for sera that were treated to dissociate immune complexes. Nor were any follow-up specimens tested. The method has not yet been confirmed by others, but it could, theoretically, offer another approach for a small number of seemingly "seronegative" patients with Lyme disease. Typically, the same information should be obtainable by either using a sensitive serological test initially, or by repeating the sensitive test days later, at which time the antibody/antigen ratio will no longer be at the equivalent point.

CULTURING THE ORGANISM

Culture is not a practical option for screening patients. Isolation of *B. burgdorferi* from blood, joint fluid, cerebrospinal fluid (CSF) or tissue has proven to be very difficult.

THE POLYMERASE CHAIN REACTION (PCR)

The PCR is not ready for use in this area. Test results have not correlated with serological or clinical findings. However, the technique may prove very powerful in identifying minute amounts of organism-specific DNA.

ANTIBODY CAPTURE AND WESTERN BLOT

The combination of antibody capture and Western blot tests is probably the best currently available approach to the serological diagnosis of Lyme disease when characteristic erythema migrans is not present. The antibody capture procedure distinguishes IgM from IgG antibody responses. The Western blot based on the electrophoretic separation of the multiple antigens of *B. burgdorferi* provides a high degree of specificity and sensitivity. A "fingerprint" is produced that can be used to eliminate false-positive serological reactions.

References

1. Henle G, Henle W. Immunofluorescence in cells derived from Burkitt's lymphoma. *J Bacteriol* 1966; 91:1248–1256.
2. Lennette ET, Henle G, Henle W. Detection of antibodies to Epstein-Barr capsid antigen by immune adherence hemagglutination. *J Clin Microbiol* 1982; 15:69–73.

3. Reedman BM, Klein G. Cellular localization of an Epstein-Barr virus-associated complement-fixed antigen in producer and non-producer lymphoblastoid cell lines. *Int J Cancer* 1973; 11:499–520.
4. Henle G, Henle W, Klein G. Demonstration of two distinct components in the early antigen complex of Epstein-Barr virus-infected cells. *Int J Cancer* 1971; 8:272–282.
5. Henle W, Henle G, Zajac B, Pearson G, Waubke R, Scriba M. Differential reactivity of human serum with early antigens induced by Epstein-Barr virus. *Science* 1970; 169:188–190.
6. Henle W, Henle G, Horwitz CA. Epstein-Barr virus-specific diagnostic tests in infectious mononucleosis. *Hum Pathol* 1974; 5:551–565.
7. Levine P, Ebbessen P, Connelly R, Das S, Middleton M, Mestre M. Complement-fixing antibody to Epstein-Barr virus soluble antigen in populations at high and low risk for nasopharyngeal carcinoma. *Int J Cancer* 1982; 29:265–268.
8. Miller G, Niederman JC, Stitt D. Infectious mononucleosis: appearance of neutralizing antibody to Epstein-Barr virus measured by inhibition of formation of lymphoblastoid cell lines. *J Infect Dis* 1972; 125:406–413.
9. Ho M. Cytomegalovirus: biology and infection. New York: Plenum Publishing Corp, 1982.
10. Kim KS, Sapienza VJ, Chen J, Wisnieski K. Production and characterization of monoclonal antibodies specific for a glycosylated polypeptide of human CMV. *J Clin Microbiol* 1983; 18:331–343.
11. Volpi A, Whitley RJ, Ceballos R, Stagno S, Pereira L. Rapid diagnosis of pneumonia due to CMV and specific monoclonal antibodies. *J Infect Dis* 1983; 147:1119–1120.
12. Gleaves CA, Smith TF, Shuster EA, Pearson GR. Rapid detection of CMV in MRC-5 cells inoculated with urine specimens by using low-speed centrifugation and monoclonal antibody to an early antigen. *J Clin Microbiol* 1984, 19:917–919.
13. Kaufman L. Serodiagnosis of fungal diseases. In Rose NR, Friedman H (eds.), *Manual of Clinical Immunology*, 2nd ed., pp 553–572. Washington DC: American Society for Microbiology, 1980.
14. de Repentigny L, Reiss E. Current trends in immunodiagnosis of candidiasis and aspergillosis. *Rev Infect Dis* 1984; 6:301.
15. Shrestka M, Grodzicki RL, Steere AC. Diagnosing early Lyme disease. *Am J Med* 1985; 78:235.

· 13 ·

Laboratory Diagnostic Assays for Autoimmune Diseases

Lewis L. Perelmutter, Ph.D.

Autoimmune diseases can be separated broadly into two categories. One group is characterized by the presence of autoantibodies that are broadly reactive with unclear or cytoplasmic antigens that do not demonstrate any tissue specificity. Included in this group are diseases such as rheumatoid arthritis, systemic lupus erythematosus (SLE), mixed connective tissue disease, scleroderma, Sjögren's syndrome and dermatomyositis/polymyositis. The second group of autoimmune diseases is characterized by autoantibodies that demonstrate tissue specificity. These diseases include thyroiditis, chronic liver diseases (including primary biliary cirrhosis and chronic active hepatitis), certain cases of pernicious anemia, and myasthenia gravis. This chapter will describe procedures for detecting autoantibodies belonging to these two broad categories.

Immunofluorescent Antinuclear Antibody Tests

The detection of circulating antibodies to nuclear antigens is an important tool in the investigation of systemic rheumatic diseases. Many techniques have been developed to detect antinuclear antibodies (ANA), but the fluorescent-ANA (FANA) test continues to be the most widely used and accepted.[1,2] Many laboratories use this test to screen sera before other techniques (such as hemagglutination, immunodiffusion, counterimmuno-electrophoresis, radioimmunoassay, and enzyme immunoassays) are used to define antibody specificity.[3] Compared with these more elaborate techniques, the FANA test has the advantages of sensitivity, reproducibility, and relative ease of performance.[4,5] A wide range of ANA are detected by this technique because most nuclear antigens are represented in carefully prepared tissue substrates.[5–7] The ANA of patients with systemic rheumatic diseases are not restricted by tissue specificity and will therefore bind to nuclear components from various species. Exceptions to this rule include sera that react specifically with human leukocyte nuclei and to Sjögren's syndrome antigens (A(SS-A/Ro)).

The major reason for ordering the FANA test is to confirm the clinical diagnosis of a systemic rheumatic disease, such as SLE. A negative FANA test does not rule out the diagnosis of SLE, but alternative diagnoses should be considered. In addition, patients receiving a drug such as procainamide, phenytoin, or hydralazine should be tested if symptoms occur suggesting a diagnosis of drug-induced SLE.[3,7]

Thus, when systemic rheumatic diseases are clinically suspected, laboratory tests for ANA should be performed. The FANA is the test of choice as it detects the presence of autoantibodies to a wide variety of nuclear and cytoplasmic antigens. If the immunofluorescence test is positive, follow-up procedures, such as immunodiffusion and radioimmunoassay, are recommended for the quantitation and identification of specific types of ANA. If the FANA test is negative and the clinical picture suggests systemic sclerosis, polymyositis, rheumatoid arthritis, or Sjögren's syndrome, alternative substrates, such as cell cultures known to contain unique antigens, should be used.

Crithidia Luciliae *Immunofluorescence Test for Antibodies to DNA*

Antibodies to DNA were initially detected in sera of patients with SLE, and their unique relationship to this disease was immediately apparent. However, it has also become evident that DNA is a molecule with multiple epitopes and that antibodies to DNA may include a heterogeneous group of immunoglobulins with a variety of specificities. Probably most common among the various antibodies reactive with DNA are those directed against antigenic determinants found in single-stranded DNA (purine and pyrimidine nucleotide determinants). Detection of such antibodies has little diagnostic specificity; they are found in a wide variety of autoimmune and connective tissue diseases. In contrast, antibodies reactive primarily or exclusively with native, double-stranded DNA manifest a remarkable association with SLE.

A source of native DNA that has proved useful for detection of anti-DNA in the clinical setting is that contained in the hemoflagellate, *Crithidia luciliae*.[8] This organism contains a modified giant mitochondrion, the kinetoplast, which contains a large concentration of well-characterized, double-stranded DNA in a stable, circular configuration. Kinetoplast DNA is unassociated with RNA or nuclear proteins. *C. luciliae* is nonpathogenic for humans and can be maintained easily in continuous culture. This technique has thus provided a simple and convenient substrate for detection of anti-DNA by an indirect immunofluorescence assay, obviating the need for chemical purification of the DNA. This method has the advantage of permitting detection of the immunoglobulin class and complement-fixing activity of antibodies to DNA using specific antisera. Thus this method has been widely adopted for routine clinical use.

ELISA for Anti-DNA and Antihistone Antibodies

The presence of antihistone antibodies can be used to verify a diagnosis of lupus induced by such drugs as procainamide and hydralazine. Antihistone antibodies can be assayed by the modified IF method with histone-reconstituted mouse kidney sections or by enzyme-linked immunosorbent assay (ELISA). The immunofluorescent (IF) method is sensitive and specific for antihistone antibodies in patients with procainamide-induced lupus. However, sera from patients with hydralazine-induced lupus often are false-negative by this method and the assay is cumbersome and expensive to perform because of the requirement of these substrate preparations. ELISA with total histones as the screening antigen detects antibodies of the wide specificities encountered in drug-induced and idiopathic SLE and is, therefore, preferable.[9]

Immunodiffusion Assays for Antibodies to Nonhistone Nuclear Antigens

As already discussed, the routine indirect immunofluorescence ANA (FANA) is the common screening test for ANA. If the FANA is positive for ANA, it is important to determine the immunologic specificity of the ANA. For example, detection of an antibody specificity to Sm antigen would be considered an important diagnostic criteria for SLE.[10] Antibody to Scl-70 antigen detected in a patient with idiopathic Raynaud's phenomenon would strongly suggest that this patient might progress to the full clinical picture of scleroderma. Thus, taking the FANA a step further and determining the immunologic specificities of the ANA may have diagnostic as well as prognostic significance.

Several methods may be used to detect immunoglobulin specificities of ANA. Indirect immunofluorescence, hemagglutination, counterimmuno-electrophonesis, immunodiffusion and ELISA have all been used under various circumstances. At present, the double immunodiffusion Ouchterlony technique is the most widely employed. Because of the growing number of new ANA specificities described, it provides the easiest way to differentiate the various immunologic specificities. The Ouchterlony technique is a very specific assay, but it does not have the sensitivity of some of the other assays, such as the ELISA. However, it still has the advantage over ELISA of not requiring purified antigens for performance of the study. Table 13–1 shows ANA specificities detectable by immunodiffusion. The table lists the antibody type, disease association and the antigen source used to detect the specific antibody. An extended review of this subject is found by Wilson and Nitsche.[11]

Autoantibodies to Small Nuclear Ribonuclear Proteins and Small Cytoplasmic Ribonucleoproteins

Antinuclear antibodies may be classified biochemically according to whether they bind a nucleic acid, a chromatin component such as a histone, a ribonucleoprotein (RNP), or some other nuclear constituent. Antibodies within each class can be detected readily in assays based on immunofluorescence. However, precise determination of the specificity of these antibodies has generally required the use of biochemically purified antigens or defined control sera for seeking lines of identity in immunodiffusion assays.

Recently, Lerner et al[12] developed an assay for autoantibodies to RNPs based on the electrophoretic identification of immunoprecipitated RNA molecules.[12] This assay provides a powerful approach for identifying nearly the entire range of autoantibodies to different RNPs, such as small nuclear RNPs (snRNPs) and small cytoplasmic RNPs (scRNPs). Compared with immunodiffusion and hemagglutination methods, the electrophoretic assay has ad-

Table 13–1   ANA Specificities Detectable by Immunodiffusion

ANTIBODY TYPE	DISEASE ASSOCIATION	ANTIGEN EXTRACT*	CONCN (mg/ml)
Sm	SLE marker	RTE	15
U-1-RNP (n-RNP)	MCTD marker if alone and with a high titer	RTE	15
SS-A/R$_o$	SS, SLE	HSE, HLE	15
SS-B/La	SS, SLE	RTE	15
Scl-70	Scleroderma	RTE	30
Jo-1	Polymyositis	RTE	30
PM-1	Polymyositis	RTE	15
PCNA	SLE	RTE	15
RANA	RA	Wil$_2$ Ext	22
MA	SLE	RTE	15

*HSE, Human spleen extract; HLE, human lymphocyte extract; Wil$_2$ Ext, Wil$_2$ cell extract (which is a human lymphoblastoid cell culture line); RTE, rabbit thymus extract.

vantages in sensitivity and ability to readily discriminate a broad range of different autoantibodies. Although the results are only semiquantitative, the levels of antibodies to most RNPs appear to fluctuate relatively little, even during exacerbations and remissions of disease activity, and antibody titer may be less important than information about the presence or absence of specific antibodies.

The different RNP autoantigens have been recognized. In general, the epitopes on each of these antigenic particles reside on one or more of the associated proteins, whereas the RNA components provide the basis for electrophoretic identification. The proteins themselves exhibit great precision when they form complexes with their RNA counterparts. Some of these proteins appear to be closely related structurally—at least they share certain antigenic conformations—and some associate with more than a single type of small RNA. For example, a monoclonal anti-Sm antibody binds both the B and D polypeptides that are shared among all of the U series of snRNPs except U3. Other polypeptides are restricted in their binding to a single type of RNA such as the 68-kilodalton (kDa) A and C polypeptides found only on the U2 snRNP or the A′ polypeptide found only on the U2 snRNP. In other words, the general nature of this system is that different antibodies are binding different proteins that complex with specific RNAs with great precision.

Identification of the different antibodies can be helpful clinically.[7,13] For example, anti-Sm antibodies are now accepted as a specific marker for systemic lupus erythematosus. On the other hand, a strong autoimmune response limited to the U1 RNP particle characterizes (but is by no means limited to) patients with mixed connective tissue disease. Similarly anti-La antibodies usually occur with anti-Ro antibodies. These antibodies are found in patients with systemic lupus erythematosus and Sjögren's syndrome. However, the Ro antibody which binds an scdRNP[14] may be the only autoantibody present in at least some patients with antinuclear-antibody-negative lupus. The Ro antibody has been linked with photosensitivity in patients who have systemic lupus erythematosus and with mothers who give birth to infants having congenital heart block. Anti-Jo 1 antibodies are currently thought to occur mainly in patients with polymyositis.[15] Finally, this assay can help discriminate spontaneous lupus from drug-induced lupus, since antibodies to native DNA and RNPs are generally not observed in the latter condition but occur in some form in the majority of patients with spontaneous lupus.[7]

Tests for Detection of Rheumatoid Factors

Rheumatoid factor is most frequently utilized to facilitate the differentiation of rheumatoid arthritis from other chronic inflammatory arthritides. Rheumatoid factor may also play an ancillary diagnostic role. Thus, it may aid in substantiating the existence of an immunologically mediated disease in a patient presenting with a disorder characterized by autoimmunity or chronic inflammation (SLE or subacute bacterial endocarditis, respectively).

Rheumatoid factors represent a group of immunoglobulins singularly characterized by their ability to react with antigenic determinants present on the Fc portion of the immunoglobulin G (IgG) molecule. After the discovery by Waaler[16] and the independent rediscovery by Rose and co-workers[17] that the sera from patients with rheumatoid arthritis agglutinated sheep erythrocytes coated with rabbit antisheep erythrocyte antibody, it was soon found that the serum factor responsible for the agglutination was a high-molecular-weight immunoglobulin of the IgM class. Numerous tests have since been devised to detect rheumatoid factor activity.

The earliest tests, and those still most widely used clinically, rely on the agglutinating properties of the IgM class of rheumatoid factors. IgG, usually human or rabbit, is bound to particulate carrier, and the presence of rheumatic factor is then recognized by agglutination or flocculation of the respective indicator system. Carrier particles frequently used include erythrocytes, latex, charcoal, and bentonite. The test systems to be described here include the latex slide agglutination and the latex tube dilution methods of Singer and Plotz.[18] These tests employ Cohn fraction II as the source of IgG antigen.

Recent promising tests for the assay of rheumatoid factor have utilized automated systems which detect changes in light-scattering properties of aggregated IgG when exposed to sera containing rheumatoid factor. These tests include laser nephelometry and rate nephelometry. These assays will not be described here but have been found to be equally sensitive and specific as and more reproducible than the more established quantitative agglutination tests. Information on these systems is available from the manufacturers.*

Rheumatoid factors may exist as the mu, gamma, alpha, and epsilon isotypes. Efforts to measure nonagglutinating rheumatoid factors have usually employed double-antibody methods, in which IgG is bound to a solid phase, usually a microtiter well, and then, after nonbound IgG is washed off, sequentially exposed, first to serum suspected of containing rheumatoid factor, and second to a purified alloantibody directed against the desired human isotype. The second antibody is radio-iodinated (radioimmunoassay) or attached to an enzyme (enzyme-linked immunosorbent assay [ELISA]). The level of rheumatoid factor in the serum is proportional to the radioactivity as measured in a gamma counter (radioimmunoassay) or to the degree of color change in the well when the developing reagent substrate is added and the light absorption is measured in a spectrophotometer at 405 nm (ELISA).

---

*Laser nephelometry, the Hyland Laser Nephelometer PDG Instrument from Hyland Laboratories, Inc., Costa Mesa, California; for rate nephelometry, the Immuno-Chemistry System ["ICS"] from Beckman Instruments, Inc., Fullerton, Calif.

Antibodies to Tissue-Specific Endocrine, Gastrointestinal and Neurological Antigens

Autoimmune diseases, those conditions in which structural or functional damage, or both, is produced by humoral and cell-mediated immune reactions with normal components of the body, may be classified as "tissue-specific" ("organ specific") or "generalized" ("non-organ specific"). The first group of diseases, comprising chronic lymphocytic thyroiditis, myasthenia gravis, pemphigus vulgaris, and others is characterized by autoimmune responses to tissue- or organ-specific antigens, antigens present in only one particular tissue or organ. The second group of diseases, which includes SLE, scleroderma, and others, is distinguished by an autoimmune response to antigens common to various organs and tissues, such as nuclear antigens.

Even though autoimmune responses to tissue-specific antigens may be both humoral and cell-mediated; at present the former responses have greater diagnostic value. The methods used to detect circulating antibodies to various tissue-specific (endocrine, gastrointestinal, and neurological) antigens are discussed below.

Antibodies to Thyroid-Specific Antigens

Sera from patients with chronic thyroiditis (Hashimoto's disease) may contain several types of antibody to thyroid antigens. Antibodies to thyroglobulin or to microsomal antigen of the thyroid are most commonly detected by routine diagnostic procedures; antibodies to the colloid antigen and cytotoxic antibodies to antigens of the thyroid cell surface are less frequently observed. In addition to being found in cases of chronic thyroiditis, these antibodies may be found with other thyroid disorders, such as primary myxedema, hyperthyroidism, colloid goiter, modular goiter, and thyroid tumors. Thyroid antibodies have also been observed in sera of patients with pernicious anemia, adrenal insufficiency, and diabetes mellitus.

Antibodies to Thyroglobulin

Thyroglobulin antibodies can be demonstrated by several procedures, such as precipitation in agar, indirect immunofluorescence, passive agglutination of cells coated with thyroglobulin, RIA, and ELISA. The newly developed ELISAs are highly sensitive and have the best performance characteristics.

Antibodies to Adrenal Antigens

Patients with idiopathic Addison's disease have circulating antibodies to adrenal antigens. The indirect IF is the most commonly used method to detect adrenal antibodies.

Table 13–2   Methods of Detection of Antibodies
to Various Tissue-Specific Antigens

ANTIGEN	DISEASE	METHOD
Parathyroid	Hypoparathyroidism	Immunofluorescent
Mitochondrial	Biliary cirrhosis	Immunofluorescent
Smooth muscle	Chronic active hepatitis	Immunofluorescent
Gastric perietal cells	Pernicious anemia	Immunofluorescent
		Complement fixation
		Radioimmunoassay
Acetylcholine receptors	Myasthenia gravis	Complement fixation
		Radioimmunoassay
		Passive hemagglutination

Antibodies to Antigens of Ovary, Testis, and Placenta

Antibodies staining the cytoplasm of cells of the theca internal interstitial and corpus luteum cells of the ovary, interstitial cells of the testis and the trophoblast of placenta have been detected in the sera of patients with Addison's disease and patients with premature ovarian failure. The antigens involved have not been very well characterized and the test itself is more of research than of diagnostic interest.

Other important antibodies to various tissue-specific antigens are listed in Table 13–2.

Concluding Remarks

Because of the size of the subject in this chapter, there are a number of important autoimmune diseases that have not been discussed. These are cardiovascular (including rheumatic fever), autoimmune hemolytic anemia, immunological platelet disorders, autoimmune reactions to blood groups (including hemolytic disease of the newborn), diabetes mellitus, renal disease, and demyelinating diseases of the central and peripheral nervous systems. A description of the pathophysiology and laboratory diagnosis can be found in Sampter et al.[19]

References

1. Bentner EH. Defined immunofluorescent staining. *Ann NY Acad Sci* 1972; 254:873–891.
2. Claymaet JE, Nakamura RM. Indirect immunofluorescent antinuclear antibody tests: Comparison of sensitivity and specificity of different substrates. *Am J Clin Pathol* 1972; 58: 388–393.
3. McCarty GA, Valencia DW, Fritzler MJ. Tan EM, ed. *Antinuclear antibodies: Contemporary*

techniques and clinical applications to connective tissue diseases. New York: Oxford University Press, 1984.

4. Molden DP, Nakamura RM, Tan EM. Standardization of the immunofluorescent test for autoantibody to nuclear antigens (ANA). Use of reference sera of defined antibody specificity. *Am J Clin Pathol* 1984; 82:47–66.

5. Nakamura RM, Peebles CL, Molden DP, Tan EM. Advances in laboratory tests for autoantibodies to nuclear antigens in systemic rheumatic diseases. *Lab Med* 1984; 15:190–198.

6. Notman DD, Kurata D, Tan EM. Profiles of antinuclear antibodies in systemic rheumatic diseases. *Ann Intern Med* 1975; 83:464–469.

7. Tan EM. Autoantibodies to nuclear antigens (ANA): their immunobiology and medicine. *Adv Immunol* 1982; 33:167–240.

8. Aarden LA, deGroot ER, Feltkamp TEW. Immunology of DNA. III. *Crithidia luciliae*, a simple substrate for the determination of anti-dsDNA with the immunofluorescence technique. *Ann NY Acad Sci* 1975; 254:505–515.

9. Rubin RL, Joslin FG, Tan EM. An improved ELISA for anti-native DNA by elimination of interference by anti-histone antibodies. *J Immunol Methods* 1983; 63:359–366.

10. Tan EM, Cohen AS, Fries JF, Masi AT, McShane DJ, Rothfield NF, Schaller, JG, Talal N, Winchester RJ. The 1982 revised criteria for classification of SLE. *Arthritis Rheum* 1983; 25:1271–1276.

11. Wilson MR, Nitsche JF. Immunodiffusion assays for antibodies to nonhistone nuclear antigens. In Rose NR, Friedman H, Fahey JL, eds. *Manual of Clinical Laboratory Immunology,* 3rd ed. Washington DC: *Amer Soc. Microbiol* 1986; 750–754.

12. Lerner EA, Lerner MR, Janeway CA Jr, Steitz JA. Monoclonal antibodies to nucleic acid-containing cellular constituents: Probes for molecular biology and autoimmune disease. *Proc Natl Acad Sci USA* 1981; 78:2737–2741.

13. Hardin JA. New approaches for analysis of antinuclear antibodies in rheumatic diseases: Etiologic insights and clinical implications. *MediLab* 1984; 1:71–74.

14. Wolin SL, Steitz JA. The Ro small cytoplasmic ribonucleoproteins: Identification of the antigenic protein and its binding site on the Ro RNAs. *Proc Natl Acad Sci USA* 1984; 81:1996–2000.

15. Mathews, MB, Bernstein RM. Myositis autoantibody inhibits histidyl-tRNA synthetase: A model for autoimmunity. *Nature* 1983; 304:177–179.

16. Waaler E. On the occurrence of a factor in human serum activating the specific agglutination of sheep blood corpuscles. *Acta Pathol Microbiol Scand* 1940; 17:172–178.

17. Rose HM, Ragan C, Pearce E, Lipmann MO. Differential agglutination of normal and sensitized sheep erythrocytes by sera of patients with rheumatoid arthritis. *Proc Soc Exp Biol Med* 1948; 68:1–11.

18. Singer JM, Plotz CM. The latex fixation test. I. Application to the serologic diagnosis of rheumatoid arthritis. *Am J Med* 1956; 21:888–892.

19. Sampter M, Talmage DW, Frank MM, Austen KF, Claman HN, eds. *Immunological Diseases,* 4th ed. Boston: Little Brown and Company, 1988.

· 14 ·

Quality Control and Quality Assurance in the Physician's Office Laboratory

ROSEMARY ALDEN, R.N., M.S., A.S.O.A.T.
IVOR EMANUEL, M.D.
MAURICE L. PEROU, M.D., F.A.C.P., F.A.S.C.P.

Although quality control did not become a way of life in the clinical laboratory until 1967 (Clinical Laboratory Improvement Act [CLIA] of 1967), the principles of quality control, based on accepted chemical practices, and derived from sound and tried statistical methods, were already well known and were being employed by most laboratories, both hospital-based and independent. During this period, physician office laboratories (POLS) were left to fend for themselves and did not have to measure up to the standards of the larger clinical laboratories. The Clinical Laboratory Improvement Amendment of 1988 (CLIA '88) forever changed the way physician office laboratories manage themselves and run their tests. The CLIA '88 regulations will, no doubt, undergo many changes, and will eventually be replaced by another set of regulations. However, the benefit of these regulations is that their basic concepts will remain as the cornerstone of good laboratory practice. This chapter has been designed to provide both educational and practical information for those who manage a POL.

Quality Control and Quality Assurance in the POL

In the past, quality control and quality assurance were synonymous and were often used interchangeably. Starting in the mid 1980s, under the persistent influence of the College of American Pathologists (CAP), the American Society of Clinical Pathologists (ASCP), and the Joint Commission of Accreditation of Hospitals (JCAHO), it has become fashionable to separate them. We think that this distinction is useful and will adhere to it.

The JCAHO defines quality control as "A systematic group of activities that recognizes errors and assures that laboratory test results are correct." As a corollary, it should be added that errors should be detected early enough so that incorrect results are not reported. Quality control, as discussed here, is composed of both internal and external quality control. The latter is often assumed to be in the domain of quality assurance. However, we prefer to limit quality assurance to "The correlation of appropriate test doing with patient care modeling as advocated by the JCAHO." (REF 2a)

Quality Control

Internal Quality Control

The purpose of internal quality control in the laboratory is to assess day-to-day performance, to identify problems as they arise, and to take corrective actions when necessary. All of these steps must, of course, be properly documented. Internal quality control has to do with the specimen and the test.

THE SPECIMEN

The specimen should be properly collected, transported, identified, and, when indicated, prepared for testing. The method of choosing the proper sample in regard to location, time, preparation, and type of population or individual should be clearly indicated and specified.

THE TEST

The more complex stage of any laboratory procedure is the performance of the test itself. This requires the following: (1) a good and up-to-date procedure manual; (2) adequately maintained equipment; (3) good record keeping; (4) good control; and (5) competent and qualified laboratory personnel from the lowest to the highest echelon.

(1) Procedure Manual. Each laboratory must have a complete procedure manual that is in accordance with federal, state, local, and public health regulations. Each new procedure should be reviewed and signed or initialed by the department head or laboratory supervisor as well as the physician in charge. This physician must be properly qualified to be the director of the laboratory

and accredited by the necessary regulatory agencies for the test or tests that are being performed under his/her directorship. Likewise, the department head, supervisor, or any other technologist initialing and/or performing the tests listed in the procedure manual must be properly qualified. The procedure manual should be reviewed in its entirety yearly by the physician in charge, who must initial the manual after reviewing it.

(2) Equipment. All equipment and instrumentation should have a well-planned and comprehensive maintenance program, which includes periodic inspections and checks. Each instrument should have its own individual file or maintenance program including records, service schedules, contracts (if any), warranties, list of inspection points, as well as frequency of inspection and checks. The records should include (1) product name, serial number, date of purchase, and initial cost; (2) points checked; (3) how frequently (weekly, monthly, etc.) the instrument was checked; (4) the past and present performance of the instrument as gauged by established parameters; and (5) records of all corrective measures taken to restore accuracy and precision as well as associated costs and time spent on correction and restoration. It would also be wise to keep any documentation of training programs that were offered with the instrument, with the maintenance records.

(3) Record Keeping. This comprises log or entry books and contains the time specimens are received, and when tests are performed and reports are issued; any information pertinent to employees; Continuing Medical Education programs, etc. One cannot emphasize enough the need for prompt, pertinent, accurate, honest, and legible record keeping. These records are the documents to which everyone refers and upon which everyone relies not only for medical, but also for legal purposes.

(4) Control. To monitor the precision and accuracy of any test system and hence assess its laboratory performance, so called "controls" are used. These controls are made up from known materials or substances and, whenever indicated, are used with each run of a given test. In addition, for certain procedures, each test sample should be checked by performance of replicates (two or more) so that statistically valid results can be obtained. The purpose of the controls is to help the analyst or technologist decide whether or not the system being used produces the expected results. Such controls can be specimens from patients, commercially known preparations (chemical or biological), randomized duplicate patient specimens, etc. Assay controls are usually sold separately from the test kits. This enables the laboratory to purchase a sufficient amount of a single lot number of the controls to last for the long periods necessary for gathering statistical data and establishing ranges. These controls help to assure accuracy, precision, and reliability of the procedures being performed. Ideally, the analytical variance should not exceed one-fourth of the physiological or biologic variance and should always

be large enough to assure optimal clinical utility. In regard to "Reagent Controls," it is recommended that new reagents be checked against old reagents before changing over to the new ones.

(5) Qualification and Goals. There should be a complete and up-to-date personnel file documenting the qualifications of each member of the laboratory. Continuing medical education should be required above and beyond the necessary requirements for accreditation, licensing, etc. A goal in the laboratory should be a constant dedication to integrity, honesty, hard work, and "the pursuit of excellence."

Terminology

After years of trial and error, various methods and techniques, based primarily on statistical analysis, have been developed that allow laboratories to monitor their daily activities and help them prevent, recognize, avoid, and correct errors, while also assuring a reasonable degree of accuracy, precision, and reliability of the laboratory tests they perform. Before these methods are discussed, it is necessary to have a clear understanding of the terminology used in the laboratory.[2]

Accuracy: True value; the closeness with which a measurement comes to the true or accepted value.

Average: See "mean."

Coefficient of variation: A calculated value for comparing the relative variability between different sets of data. This measure allows a practical comparison of standard deviation values by expressing them as a percentage of the mean value (Fig. 14–1).

Confidence level: ±2 SDs from the mean; 95% of all values fall into this range.

CV Formula

$$CV = \frac{SD}{\overline{X}} \times 100$$

CV = Coefficient of variation

SD = standard deviation

$\overline{X}$ = mean

Figure 14–1.   Coefficient of Variation.

Control serum: A serum with a known concentration of the same constituents as those being determined in the patient sample.

Gaussian curve: A graph plotting the distribution of values around the mean; normal frequency curve (Fig. 14–2).

Levy-Jennings chart: A quality control chart that demonstrates the precision of a method. It is a simple way of displaying control data graphically. By doing so, it provides a visual indication of where errors have occurred or might have occurred (Figs. 14–3 to 14–8).

Mean: The figure obtained when the sum of a set of values is divided by the number of values; the average. This is an arithmetic average of control test values observed over a period of time, commonly used to measure accuracy. The mean establishes a benchmark against which the accuracy of an individual test control result can be compared.

Normal value: This term is used, not in reference to a state of good health, or to a Gaussian distribution, but strictly in the concept of reference values, that is, a set of values of a measured quality obtained either from a group of individuals or a single individual, who were presumably healthy.

Outlier: A value outside of ±2 SDs.

Population: The entire group of items or individuals from which samples under consideration are presumed to have come.

Gaussian Curve

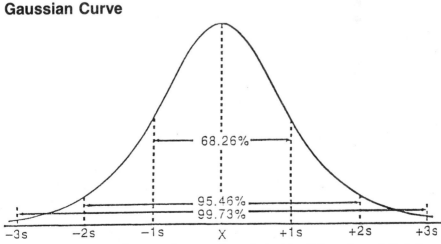

Figure 14–2. If the total area under curve is equivalent to all the values plotted, then we can expect the following: 1) 68.26% of the test values will be within ±1 SD; 2) 95.46% of the test values will be within ±2 SD; 3) 99.73% of the test values will be within ±3 SD.

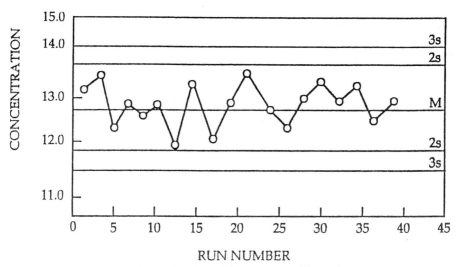

Figure 14–3. Levey-Jennings Chart. Acceptable performance.

Precision: The reproducibility of results; the closeness of obtained values to each other. A method is said to be precise when the values obtained are consistently reproducible. Precision can be expressed mathematically, by the standard deviation (SD), or coefficient of variation (CV). One can nevertheless achieve precision without accuracy (Table 14–1).

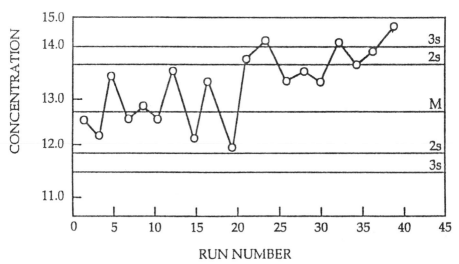

Figure 14–4. Levey-Jennings Chart. Shift upward of the mean.

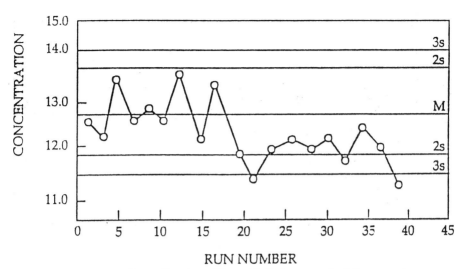

Figure 14–5. Levey-Jennings Chart. Shift downward of the mean.

Random Error: An error whose source cannot be definitely identified. When one falls outside the ±2 SD limit, it may be due to chance.

Reliability: Accuracy plus precision. It means reproducibility, the extent to which a statistically derived measure from a sample gives the same results upon repeated sampling under identical conditions.

Sample: In statistics, a subgroup of a population.

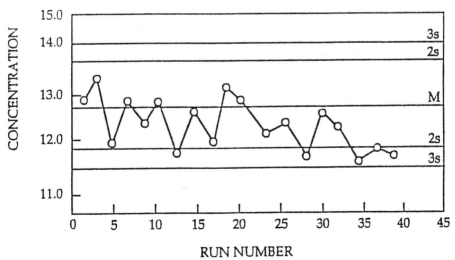

Figure 14–6. Levey-Jennnigs Chart. Trend/drift downward of the mean.

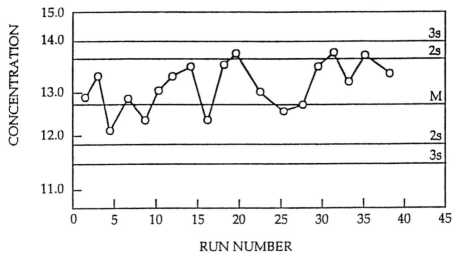

Figure 14–7.   Levey-Jennings Chart. Trend/drift upward of the mean.

Sensitivity: The minimum reportable result, or the lowest true positive result that can be detected (the positivity of disease).

Specificity: Proportion of negative results among patients without the disease (the negativity of health).

Shift: An indication of error in the analysis, detected by a continuing series of values above or below the mean (see Figs. 14–4 and 14–5). A shift is especially significant when it occurs outside the standard deviation limits. It may reflect a significant change in reagents, equipment, or environment.

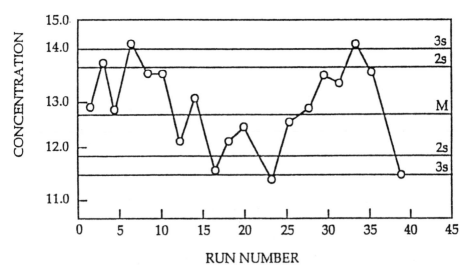

Figure 14–8.   Levey-Jennings Chart. Loss of precision.

Table 14–1   Comparison of Achieving
Precision Without Accuracy*

| | GLUCOSE (110 mg/dl) | |
	Lab A	Lab B
	90 mg/dl	111 mg/dl
	91	109
	92	112
	88	110
	90	110
	89	108
	90	111
	92	108
	90	112
	88	108
MEAN	90 mg/dl	110 mg/dl
	± 1 S.D. = 1.4	± 1 S.D. = 1.5

*Lab A and Lab B both have excellent precision, noted by their small S.D. They are able to reproduce virtually the same results day-in and day-out. However, the target value is 110 mg/dl, so therefore, Lab B is the only one with Accuracy and Precision; Lab A only has Precision.

Standard: A chemical solution whose exact concentration is known and can be used as a reference or calibration substance. They have been divided into primary standards, secondary standards, and standard reference materials.

Primary standards are highly purified chemicals that can be directly weighed or measured to produce a solution whose concentration is exactly known. These chemicals may be weighed directly for the preparation of solutions of selected concentration or for the standardization of solutions of unknown strength. Companies supply primary standards with certificates of analysis for each lot. They are generally used as "calibrating standards."

Secondary standards, according to Tietz, are "solutions whose concentration cannot be exactly known by weighing the solute and dissolving a known amount into a volume of solution." He adds, "the concentration of secondary standards is usually determined by analysis of an aliquot of the solution by an acceptable reference method," by use of a primary standard to calibrate the method. These standards are either "in-house" or commercially prepared, and are used in the day-to-day analyses. Besides the chemical secondary standards described above, there is another type of secondary standard represented by biological materials or substances such as pools of sera processed for stability and with certain substances added to raise constituents to desired levels.

Standard reference materials (SRM's): There are certified reference materials available from the National Bureau of Standards. They are prepared and used for three main purposes: (1) to help develop accurate methods of analysis, known also as reference methods; (2) for calibration; and (3) to assure adequacy and integrity of measurement in quality assurance programs.

In summary one can say that a standard serves as a measure or model to which other similar substances or materials should compare and conform. Let us emphasize that controls, as opposed to standards, are specimens of solutions that are analyzed solely for quality control purposes and are never used for calibration purposes.

Standard deviation: The measure of the spread of a population of values around the mean. It focuses on test control results by indicating how much individual test values vary above or below the mean value. The greater the standard deviation (i.e., the spread of values), the greater the difference between individual test results and the less precision there is in the procedure. A range of one standard deviation below the mean to one standard deviation above the mean encompasses approximately 68% of the test values, with half of the values on each side of the mean. Acceptable limits for most assays are two standard deviations above and below the mean, which will include 95% of the test values.

Statistics: The science of collecting and classifying facts in order to show their significance.

Systematic error: A variation that may influence results to be consistently higher or lower than the real value.

Trend (or drift): An indication of error in the analysis, detected by an ever increasing value in the control samples, which is a series of six values that increase or decrease on consecutive days (see Figures 14–6 and 14–7). A trend or drift away from the mean becomes apparent on the Levy-Jennings chart. A trend is usually an indication of a deterioration in reagents, including enzyme reagents and quality control samples, or results from improper or faulty storage temperature.[3]

Validity (efficacy or efficiency): The measure of the actual practical value of the diagnostic data in regard to the benefits (in relation to solving clinical problems) versus the risks and costs of the test.

Westgard rules: Specific limits on how much error is allowed in the control value before the results of a patient's tests are rejected.

Variance: A measure of the variation shown by a set of observations, the average or squared deviation from the mean; or the square of the standard deviation.

With the definitions out of the way, let us now discuss some of the statistical control techniques mentioned above.

Statistical Control Techniques

Test results do not have to be 100% precise or 100% accurate in order to provide meaningful results that will aid the physician's diagnosis. However, specific upper and lower limits must be set for how much error can be allowed in tests. Results exceeding those limits must be analyzed in an effort to determine whether test procedures are "in control" or "out of control." The limits of test reliability are determined by calculation of quality control statistics, specifically the techniques used for the general evaluation of the mean, standard deviation, and coefficient of variation; the establishment of "normals;" the use of predictive value, control charts, trend analysis of variance technique, pattern recognition, Youden plot, and other methods. Each particular discipline (chemical, biological, method verification) must select the statistical control techniques best devised to suit its purpose.

In the following paragraphs we will discuss Levy-Jennings charts, systematic errors, random errors, as well as some fallacies of quality control and method verification.

The Levy-Jennings Chart is a visual representation of the distribution of the control values, which when correctly performed and maintained, will provide visual indications of where errors have occurred, or might occur. The Levy-Jennings charts are permanent records and must be kept current at all times for measurement of day-to-day laboratory performance. It is also good laboratory practice that they be displayed or at least readily available.

The following section explains how to compute the statistics for the Levy-Jennings charts. It further demonstrates how to plot the charts on graph paper for easy visual comparisons, and how to interpret them. The techniques described apply only to procedures in which controls are run concurrently with patient samples so that benchmarks are established for accuracy and precision.

Ideally, at least 20 determinations should be run to provide values for standard deviation calculations. However, preliminary data may be generated with as few as 11 determinations.[1]

BEGINNING THE LEVY-JENNINGS CHART

Initially, the mean acceptable control ranges used are those assigned by the manufacturer. Obtain any size and dimension of linear graph paper.

1. Locate the middle line on the left side of the graph paper.
2. Find the "mean value" for the control serum (listed on the vial itself or in the package insert).
3. Write this value opposite the middle line on the left side of the graph paper and draw a heavy line across the chart to indicate the mean value.
4. Obtain the minimum acceptable value for the control serum (two standard deviations below the mean). Count down an appropriate number of lines below the mean value and write this value on the left side of the

graph next to the appropriate line. Draw a dotted line from this point across the chart; this will represent the lowest acceptable control value.

5. Obtain the maximum acceptable value for the control serum (two standard deviations above the mean) as above. From the mean value line, count up an appropriate number of lines and write this value on the left side of the graph next to the appropriate line. Draw a dotted line from this point across the chart. This will represent the highest acceptable control value.

PLOTTING THE FIRST 11 CONTROL VALUES (AS APPLIED TO THE
ALLERGY LABORATORY)

For each or the first 11 assays, plot the immunoglobulin E (IgE) concentration value for the control tubes. The bold vertical lines on the graph paper should be marked with each assay run date. Assume that you run the total IgE assay 11 consecutive times and that the following average calculated concentration values were found for the total IgE control serum: 94.4, 100.5, 85.0, 97.4, 102.4, 109.0, 96.2, 88.3, 117.2, 108.0, 100.5. The following mean and range were printed on the control vial: 100 kU/l (80–120 kU/l). Two conclusions can be drawn from the above representative information:

1. All plotted values fall within the accepted upper and lower limits, indicating that the test procedures were under control.
2. Of the 11 control values obtained, six of them (54%) were above the mean value and five (46%) were below. This is another indication that the procedures were in good control.

PREPARING INTERNAL PERFORMANCE LIMITS

After 11 to 20 control data points have been collected, the performance limits as assigned by the manufacturer must be reevaluated. Internal performance limits are based on the assumption that over an extended period of time, the values for a particular lot number of control will fall in a "normal distribution," that is, that the majority of points will lie closer to the mean value (the average of all control values obtained) with fewer and fewer points falling on either side of the mean and standard deviation for control data actually obtained in your laboratory. These data will then replace the original mean and control ranges, those which were stated by the manufacturers' package insert.

Instructions are given below for manual calculation of these parameters; however, most hand calculators can perform the calculations required to determine these statistics.

An example of these calculations can be seen in Table 14–2. For each total IgE assay, enter the average value for the control serum in the column labeled "X."

To calculate the mean value, add the values in column "X." Divide their sum by the total number of assays listed and enter the results. This is the mean (or average) value for all controls you have run.

<table>
<tr><td colspan="4">Table 14–2   Calculating Internal Performance Limits
Using Standard Deviation</td><td></td></tr>
</table>

n	x	d	d2	
1	95.4	4.5	20.25	
2	100.5	0.6	0.36	x = 99.9
3	85.0	14.9	222.01	
4	97.4	2.5	6.25	1 s.d. = 9.23
5	102.4	2.5	6.25	
6	109.0	9.1	82.81	2 s.d. = 18.46
7	96.2	3.7	13.69	
8	88.3	11.6	134.56	range = 81.44 − 118.36
9	117.2	17.3	299.29	
10	108.0	8.1	65.61	
11	100.5	0.6	0.36	
12				
13			851.44	
14				
15				
16				

To calculate the standard deviation, use the sequence below:

1. Calculate the difference between each individual value listed in column "X" and the mean value. Enter the difference in the column labeled "d." Ignore the + or − designation of these differences.
2. Square each value in the column "d" (i.e., multiply each difference by itself) and record the result in the column labeled "d2."
3. Divide the sum of the "d2" column by the total number of assays listed, less one (1).
4. Calculate the square root of the number obtained in step 3 above. The value is one standard deviation (SD).
5. Multiply the SD value by 2. This value will provide the distance from the mean of both the upper (+2 SD) and lower (−2 SD) acceptable control limits.

The entire process from the section, "Beginning your Levy-Jennings Chart" should be repeated whenever there is a change in lot number of the control. **The process must be performed for each lot number of the control before that control lot is put into use in an assay from which patient results are reported.**

The gathering of data for a particular lot number of controls should be done while the previous lot number of controls is still being used. To gather data for calculation of statistics, a few samples of the control may be run as patients in an assay. It is important to run the samples in as many assays as possible, using as many lot numbers of immunoassay kits as possible. If more than one technician performs the assay, each should run the assay during this data collection process. In this way, a more accurate representation of the normal variation that occurs in the laboratory will be achieved.

The locations and patterns of the points plotted on the Levy-Jennings chart can give you significant indications of changes in the test system. Statistically, over a period of time, the plotted points should be distributed so that as many values appear above the mean as below it. However, this pattern will not necessarily occur consistently in actual performance.

Common Errors in Quality Control

RANDOM ERRORS

Random errors increase the extent of variability of results (affects precision of the method); that is, they increase the SD value, but the mean of the results is largely unaffected. These errors can be minimized, but never totally eliminated (Fig. 14–9).[4]

Types of Random Error
1. Improper sample collection.
2. Clerical errors.
3. Effect of light, evaporation, or temperature on sample.
4. Improper glassware washing.
5. Instrument malfunction.
6. Chemist error.
7. Pipettes and volumetric glassware with manufacturing variations.
8. Electronic and optical variations in instruments.
9. Variations in curvettes/microtiter plates.
10. Interference from other substances in the analyzed sample.
11. Incorrect reading of results.
12. Dilution and calculation errors.
13. Software usage of errors.
14. Lack of or improper instrument calibration.

Evaluation and Correction of Random Errors. Statistically, there is a 5% chance of a random error. Whenever the test is in control if this normal variation should occur, the appropriate action is to: (1) Reanalyze the control only (not patient samples), while holding patient results; and (2) Record both control values if the re-analyzed control now falls within accepted limits. Patient results may now be reported. Special consideration should be given to an increase in random errors.

Evaluation and Correction of Increased Random Errors. When two or more consecutive values fall outside ±2 SD limit, this is an indication that random

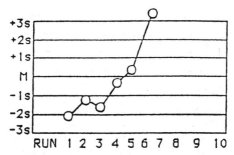

Figure 14–9. Random error. The run is considered out of control when one control value exceeds the mean ±3s. This applies within the run only.

error is increasing and the test procedure is out of control. When this occurs, all possible sources of error must be checked as follows:

1. Repeat the test using a fresh vial of control; do not report patient results.
2. If result of this control falls within range, the patient values may then be reported.
3. If the result on the fresh vial of control is still unacceptable, this is an indication that something in the test is failing. Calibrate all instruments, ensure proper pipetting technique and review the assay procedure to try to isolate the problem and restore precision and accuracy. The results of patient samples run during an out of control situation are unreliable and should be repeated. In this situation, it is not necessary to include the outlier results in the statistical calculations for the control. NOTE! DO NOT ANALYZE SPECIMENS, OR REPORT PATIENT RESULTS, until the problem is resolved. All actions taken to resolve the problem should be recorded in the record book, along with the results for the controls.

SYSTEMATIC ERRORS

Systematic errors displace the mean value in one direction, which may be up or down, but do not affect the overall variability as shown by the SD value. Non-random error affects results in a consistent manner (Fig. 14–10).

Types of Systematic Error.

1. Inaccuracy of standards
2. Instability of reagents
3. Incorrect sampling
4. Instrument malfunction

Evaluation and Correction of Westgard Rules. The specific limits on how much error is allowed in the control before the results of a patient test can be rejected are:

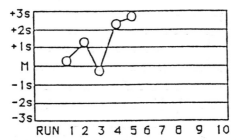

Figure 14–10. Systematic error applies within and across runs. Within the run, two consecutive control values (or 2 of 3 control values when 3 levels are being run) exceed the "same" (mean + 2s) or (mean − 2s) limit. Across runs, the previous value for a particular control level exceeds the "same" (mean + 2s) or (mean − 2s) limit.

1. Both controls are outside the ±2 SD limit.
2. One control (same concentration) is outside the ±2 SD limit in two consecutive runs.
3. Controls in four consecutive runs have value greater than ±1 SD all in the same direction.
4. 10 consecutive control values fall either above or below the mean.

If a given result falls outside the above-mentioned limits, the patient test results should automatically be rejected.

Evaluation and Correction of a Shift.

1. Check to see whether the lot number of the reagents has changed; different materials may yield different values.
2. If the shift is below the mean, check expiration dates of reagents used.
3. Check all pipette and fluorometer calibrations for the runs in question to determine whether they have been consistent.
4. Analyze pipetting techniques to determine their accuracy.
5. Calculate and plot new mean and standard deviation values if warranted.

Fallacies of Quality Control.[5]

1. Most errors occur during the analytic run.
    Contrary to a common assumption, most errors do not occur during the analytic run, but rather during the collection and processing of the specimen and in transcribing the test results to the patient report form.
2. Good performance on proficiency surveys indicates a proficient laboratory.
    Good results on proficiency surveys may or may not indicate a proficient laboratory. More often than not, samples are treated "specially"

by laboratories and are not randomly placed in the patient's test run. Some laboratories have been known to have the proficiency survey sample analyzed several times by only the "best" technologists. The mean value is determined and sent to the proficiency testing agency. This defeats the purpose of proficiency testing and is a gross-waste of the patient's money.

3. Increased accuracy and precision equal better patient care.

Increased accuracy and precision do not necessarily mean better patient care. There comes a point with every test at which increasing the accuracy and precision becomes meaningless. When this point is reached, it makes no sense to implement more costly and inconvenient methods for the sake of increased accuracy and precision. Most physicians will agree that a possible test error in a cholesterol determination of 4 or 8% will have no effect on how they evaluate a patient's condition. Does it make sense, then, to incorporate a more costly, inconvenient cholesterol method with a CV of 4% instead of an inexpensive, convenient method with a CV of 8%.

4. If abnormal and normal controls are within the established control range, are the patient test values necessarily correct?

Control samples are not treated exactly as the patient's specimen. For example, the control is not collected from a patient, is not transported to the laboratory, and is not centrifuged. For these reasons, one cannot automatically assume that all of the patient values are correct because the abnormal and normal controls are within the established control range.

Method Verification

This is a procedure mandated by CLIA '88 regulations (Federal Register, Vol. 57, No. 40, p. 7164, Section 493.1213). These regulations stipulate that any laboratory implementing a test method of either moderate or high complexity after September 1, 1992, and before September 1, 1994, MUST demonstrate that the method performs in accordance with the manufacturer's stated claims within the laboratory environment. Typically, a manufacturer assesses several performance characteristics for a method. Among these are (see terminology) accuracy, precision, sensitivity, specificity, reportable range of patient results, and reference range. The NCCLS (National Committee for Clinical Laboratory Standards) has written a simple method verification procedure.[6] A copy of the NCCLS manual should be kept in the laboratory.

SIMPLE METHOD VERIFICATION

Introduction of a new instrument or analytical method should be done with great care and deliberation. In this section, two protocols are presented for verifying that a method or system will perform as intended by the manufacturer.

1. Goals of the Simple Method Verification. The purpose of this simple procedure is to answer the following questions:

1. Is the operator sufficiently familiar with the instructions, equipment, and materials required?
2. Will the test system or assay produce accurate results when patient specimens are analyzed?
3. Can the operator adequately perform testing with the test system of the assay?

2. Familiarization Study for the Simple Method Verification. The following familiarization study should be performed to allow the operator to become familiar with the operator's manual, to practice the procedure, and to determine whether there are any problems in the following instructions:

1. Read and study the operator's manual or package insert and any training materials provided by the manufacturer:
2. Run the test system or assay on control material recommended by the manufacturer.
3. Run two levels of assayed control material whose package insert has values for this test system or assay and determine that the results of five replicates of each level fall within the manufacturer's allowable range as specified in the package insert.
4. Prepare a control chart or table to record future control values.

3. Performance Study for Simple Method Verification. The following study should be performed to verify that the test system or assay will perform satisfactorily in the office laboratory:

1. Run two levels of control specimens and five patient specimens—all in triplicate.
2. Take an aliquot of each of these specimens (patients and controls) and test by an established method in the laboratory or send to a reference laboratory for testing.
3. Add the control specimen values to control charts or tables to determine whether the method had adequate reproducibility.
4. Compare the results of the new test system or assay to the results of the established method or reference laboratory method.

External Quality Control

Internal quality control is focused on monitoring a given laboratory procedure or set of procedures strictly within the confines of the laboratory, whereas external quality control comprises methods and means used to compare the performance of various laboratories. It is thus an interlaboratory quality control or interlaboratory comparison program.

A number of professional societies, regulatory agencies, private agencies and manufacturers offer external quality control programs in one form or another. The basic tenet is that all participants analyze the same lot of material, either daily or on a regular basis (monthly, quarterly). The results after tabulation are evaluated by referees or other authoritative sources and a summary report or critique is subsequently issued. The results not only are compared and categorized, but are also subject to corrective measures. Furthermore, the results of these surveys are often sent to certain regulatory agencies for purposes of regulation and certification. This applies when repeated discrepancies or errors occur in regard to one or more procedures. External quality control programs may be regional or national, or both. In a regional program, often a group of laboratories in a given geographical area use the same lots of quality control specimens on a daily basis for their internal quality control program. On a national basis, large numbers of laboratories enroll in a specific program. Various programs and regulatory agencies are available. Some of the more important of these are discussed next.

The College of American Pathologists Proficiency Testing Program or Interlaboratory Comparison Program

This program is very comprehensive and encompasses all of the laboratory disciplines, including allergy testing. It consists of a series of surveys that are sent to participating laboratories on a regular basis. The CAP also offers to participants survey-validated reference material, which contains the same material sent to the participants in survey program shipments, and is numbered in the same manner as the survey specimen. These reference materials will help the participant define the existence of a problem and facilitate its correction. In addition, they may be of help when a new method is being devised; they may be used as a check to backup systems and alternate methods; they may be used on occasion as blind specimens and, finally, as a check on internal quality control pool material. Currently there are two groups which have proficiency testing programs for total and specific IgE. One of these is sponsored by the CAP, and the other by the Society for Internal Medicine.

Proficiency test samples for the CAP testing are sent three times a year. Each shipment includes five samples for each analyte test. A separate grading formula is established for each specialty and subspecialty. The minimum passing score, at this time, is 80%. Changes in grading procedures are expected in 1994.

The CAP also offers the "Q-Probes" in a special program that allows a laboratory to gauge and improve its quality of care through the performance of structured internal audits that enable each laboratory to be compared with other laboratories across the country on the basis of certain standards of practice. This is probably more akin to quality assurance than to quality control. Finally the CAP recently has published some excellent guidelines concerning the "categories of responses to unacceptable results." Too often in the past, the physician in charge would write some vague comments concerning these results. Now, by following the CAP guidelines, he/she can adopt these four categories: (1) methodologic problems (problems related to instruments, faulty standards or reagent, incorrect calibration); (2) technical problems (misinterpretation, misidentification, dilution error; (3) clerical errors (transcription or transportation errors); (4) problems with survey materials (specimens hemolyzed, contaminated; and (5) unexplained or unexplainable problems.

Federal Agencies have certain regulatory functions that are being greatly extended. The CDC (Centers for Disease Control), pursuant to the implementation of the Clinical Laboratories Improvement Act of 1967 (CLIA-1967), has developed a proficiency testing program for clinical laboratories involved in interstate commerce. It has also participated in cooperative standardization programs, for example, with the World Health Organization (WHO).

The Department of Health and Human Services. Since 1967, when the federal government started effectively to regulate laboratories through the Clinical Laboratory Improvement Act (CLIA 1967), this department has exerted a great and lasting influence on the practice of laboratory medicine. The new CLIA 1988 has recently been approved and is now being implemented. The latest rules and regulations are far-reaching and will greatly influence the practice of laboratory medicine in the U.S.A. for many years to come.

The National Committee for Clinical Laboratory Standards (NCCLS). This committee was chartered as a nonprofit corporation for the purpose of promoting the development of national standards for clinical laboratories, and providing a mechanism for defining and resolving problems that influence the quality of work performed. It has written comprehensive volumes pertinent to various laboratory procedures and disciplines. We have been unable so far to find any reference in their manuals to allergy testing in the laboratory.

Miscellaneous Agencies. It is imperative that all laboratories, including the Physician's Office Laboratory (POL), observe the United States Department of Labor's Occupational Safety and Health Administration (OSHA) regulations pertinent to safety, including biohazards, and that all necessary forms, biohazard stickers, and exposure control plan, are taken care of and properly displayed when indicated. Likewise, the POL should be in compliance with local fire regulations, electrical regulations, and any other pertinent regulations (relating to catastrophic events; either natural, such as hurricanes and tornadoes; or man-made, such as excessive radiation exposure). In conclusion, the new federal regulations as well as those already being implemented by many other agencies (such as CAP, ASCP, etc.) will mandate a high level of external quality control practice. Failure to attain and maintain this level may result in large fines as well as revocation of accreditation and/or license.

Quality Assurance

Quality assurance is relatively new. Until a few years ago, the Joint Commission on Accreditation of Health Care Organizations (JCAHO) professed not to evaluate the quality of the work performed in the hospital, being content to evaluate only the evidence of it, that is, the paperwork. It has now changed course and also evaluates actual patient care. Regarding the laboratory, the JCAHO states that "Quality Assurance involves correlating appropriate test choices with patient care modalities to assure high quality patient care" (The Joint Commission. Monitoring and Evaluation Series. Rober and Franberg, Ed. JCAHO, 1987, p. 7. Monitoring and Evaluation. Pathology and Medical Laboratories Services).

The quality assurance program should start by asking itself these questions: (1) Does the right patient get the right test and the right report at the right time? (2) Had the patient been properly evaluated beforehand, and is he/she going to benefit from the test? (3) Had the right test been performed correctly? (4) Had the right report been issued correctly (i.e., had the correct units of measurement been used, had the decimal points been placed where they should have been? (5) Is the patient report legible, with no mistakes, and readily available? (6) Did the clinician receive the report in time to benefit the patient?

One should start quality assurance in the same fashion as quality control: by having a complete quality assurance manual that is reviewed and updated yearly. Despite the accepted separation of quality control and quality assurance, too often articles are written and manuals are prepared which show a complete lack of understanding of the differences between the two. Let us emphasize once more that there should be no duplication between the two manuals, and that no duplication will exist if external quality control is well defined and kept separately in the quality control manual. This does not mean that proficiency surveys and the likes do not constitute an excellent form of peer review. They do, and hence they literally provide an assurance of quality. However, they are clearly outside the main confines of the JCAHO definition, which emphasizes the correlation of appropriate test choice with patient care modalities.

Scope of Quality Assurance

In accordance with the recommendations of the JCAHO and CAP, the following guidelines should be adopted and included in the official laboratory procedure manual:

1. Assign responsibility for the QA program; that is, place a person in charge. Often, the person in charge is a technologist who works very closely with the physician–director. The latter should, whenever possible, be a member of the hospital QA committee and any other appropriate committee (such as transfusion, infection control). No policy decision should be made unilaterally. At all times, the physician–director should be informed of policy changes and must approve them before they are implemented.
2. Define scope of program and identify its important goals.
3. Devise certain parameters (indicators, monitors) that will serve as a guideline for evaluation and establish thresholds.
4. Appropriateness of collection time and technique, limit on time of processing, proper identification and labeling of specimen, their acceptability, the manner and time of transmission of the tests to the attending physician and, when appropriate, to the patient should be included.
5. A plan for prompt evaluation and corrective actions should be developed. For this purpose, a problem identification and corrective action form is necessary. It will help to pinpoint the problems, justify and categorize their study, evaluate the benefits, formulate appropriate recommendations and assure followup.
6. In that connection, one should make sure that corrective actions, pertinent evaluations and problems not only are assessed, but also result in improvement in patient care. This can be done only if the data obtained are communicated to all interested parties and if the followup steps taken result in implementation of concrete measures.

Quality Assurance of Personnel

Without well-trained and quality-conscious personnel, no matter how many graphs, curves, or controls used, quality control and quality assurance will be only perfunctory, with poor-to-mediocre results that will be reflected in an overall lack of quality of the laboratory. It is imperative that, in every single laboratory, high standards for high-grade personnel be maintained, and that proper certification be required of all lab workers. Likewise, CME programs for all laboratory employees should be mandatory. These programs may be local, regional, national, or international and must be approved before proper credit can be given

In summary, the quality assurance program should consist of an ongoing review and evaluation of the quality and particularly of the appropriateness of laboratory procedures. The program should help define, monitor, improve, and hence assure the quality of laboratory performance. To this end, certain parameters should be established; appropriate documentation should be kept; actions should be taken; and finally the impact on actual patient care and clinical situations should be evaluated regularly. In addition, just as quality control can be internal and external, so can quality assurance.

Conclusion

We hope that this overview of quality control and quality assurance will acquaint the reader with the essential requirements and basic tenets for a modern clinical laboratory. Quality laboratory results do not come about just because one purchases quality reagents or equipment. It is the responsibility of every laboratory director to assure that errors do not occur in his/her laboratory. The strict scientific discipline of the general clinical laboratory will of necessity become a way of life in the POL, thus better protecting both the patient and the laboratorian. Likewise, regulations, references, and their inevitable counterpart, the regulatory agencies, will continue to exist. We believe that they are necessary. Finally, it must be remembered that the POL is of great value to patients, as it is often an advantage for the patient to have these laboratory services readily available, for better quality and cost-effectiveness.[7]

References

1. Laboratory Assurance Program. Richmond: Quality America, 1990.
2. Plaut D, Silberman J. American Dade Quality Control, American Hospital Corporation, 1984.
3. Physician Office Laboratory Manual, NCCLS Document POL2-T2, June, 1992.
4. Henry JB. *Clinical Diagnosis by Laboratory Methods*. Philadelphia: WB Saunders Company, 1976.
5. Kaplan LA, Pesce AJ. *Clinical Chemistry Theory, Analysis, and Correlation*. Philadelphia: C.V. Mosby Company, 1989.
6. Physician Office Lab Guidelines, NCCLS Document POL1-T2, June, 1992.
7. Laboratory Quality Assurance Manual. Piscataway: Kabi Pharmacia Diagnostics, 1993.

· *Index* ·

Cytoplasmic ribonuclearproteins, small, autoantibody, autoimmune disease, 127–128

Degranulation, nonimmune mast-cell, immunoglobulin E mediated disease, 6–8
Dennie-Morgan lines, *in vitro* diagnosis, primary care physician, 98
Diagnostic approaches, primary care physician, *in vitro* diagnosis, 100–103
Diet, pregnant mother's, modification of, prediction of allergic phenotype, 91
Dose, immunotherapy, RAST, based on, 68–78
Dual response, hypersensitivity reaction, immunoglobulin E mediated, allergic reaction, 4–6

Endocrine antigen, antibody, autoimmune disease, 130–131
Environmental factors, immunoglobulin E antibody, allergy prediction, 86–87
Eosinophils, immunoglobulin E mediated disease, 14
Epstein-Barr virus, 118–119

Failure, causes of, mRAST-based immunotherapy, 76
False positives, *in vitro* measurement, immunoglobulin E antibody, performance characteristics, 35–37
Fatigue syndrome, chronic, *see* Chronic fatigue syndrome
Feeding methods
breast feeding, infant, with allergic risk, 92
infant, allergic risk, 92–93
milk, to infant, with allergic risk, 92
solids, to infant, with allergic risk, 92
F/N modified RAST, skin endpoint titration, relationship to, 56–57
Food allergies, *in vitro* measurement, immunoglobulin E antibody, role in, 79–83
Fungal sinusitis, 110

Gastrointestinal antigen, autoimmune disease, antibody, 130–131

Genetic factors, allergy prediction, immunoglobulin E antibody, 86

Helper subtypes, immunoglobulin E mediated disease, 15
"High allergic risk" phenotype, prediction of, immunoglobulin E antibody, 88–91
Hypersensitivity reaction, immunoglobulin E mediated, allergic reaction
dual response, 4–6
immediate, 1–4
challenge phase, 3
sensitization phase, 2–3
late-phase reaction, 4–6

Immune dysfunctions, with chronic sinusitis, 107–111
Immunodeficiency syndrome, with chronic sinusitis, 107–110
Immunofluorescent antinucler antibody test, autoimmune disease, 124–127
Immunoglobulin E
immunologic disorder, elevated serum level of immunoglobulin E, 22
mediated disease
cyclic nucleotide, and autonomic systems, 9–11
cytokine, and allergy, 11–18
eosinophils, 14
helper subtypes, 15
hypersensitivity reactions, 1–4
immunology of, 1–19
immunomolecular biological response substances, 16, 17
inflammation, 15
late-phase reaction, dual response, 4–6
mast cell-derived mediator, 17
mast cells, 14–15
mediator release trigger, 8
nonimmune mast-cell degranulation, 6–8
T-cells, cytokine secretion, 16–17
regulation, mediated disease, 15
skin endpoint titration, *in vitro* measurement, relationship, 53–59
Immunoglobulin E antibody
allergy prediction, *in vitro* measurement, infancy, 84–96